Breast Cancer Prevention and Treatment

W0105931

Lida A. Mina • Anna Maria Storniolo
Hal Douglas Kipfer • Cindy Hunter
Kandice K. Ludwig

Breast Cancer Prevention and Treatment

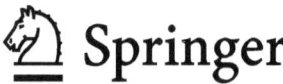 Springer

Lida A. Mina
IU Simon Cancer Center
Indiana University School of Medicine
Indianapolis, IN
USA

Cindy Hunter
Medical and Molecular Genetics Dept
Indiana University Health Physicians
Indianapolis, IN
USA

Anna Maria Storniolo
IU Simon Cancer Center
Indiana University School of Medicine
Indianapolis, IN
USA

Kandice K. Ludwig
Department of Surgery
Indiana University School of Medicine
Indianapolis, IN
USA

Hal Douglas Kipfer
Department of Radiology
Indiana Radiology Partners
Indianapolis, IN
USA

ISBN 978-3-319-19436-3   ISBN 978-3-319-19437-0   (eBook)
DOI 10.1007/978-3-319-19437-0

Library of Congress Control Number: 2016940904

© Springer International Publishing Switzerland 2016
This work is subject to copyright. All rights are reserved by the Publisher, whether the whole or part of the material is concerned, specifically the rights of translation, reprinting, reuse of illustrations, recitation, broadcasting, reproduction on microfilms or in any other physical way, and transmission or information storage and retrieval, electronic adaptation, computer software, or by similar or dissimilar methodology now known or hereafter developed.
The use of general descriptive names, registered names, trademarks, service marks, etc. in this publication does not imply, even in the absence of a specific statement, that such names are exempt from the relevant protective laws and regulations and therefore free for general use.
The publisher, the authors and the editors are safe to assume that the advice and information in this book are believed to be true and accurate at the date of publication. Neither the publisher nor the authors or the editors give a warranty, express or implied, with respect to the material contained herein or for any errors or omissions that may have been made.

Printed on acid-free paper

This Springer imprint is published by Springer Nature
The registered company is Springer International Publishing AG Switzerland

Contents

Contributors

Cindy Hunter Medical and Molecular Genetics Dept, Indiana University Health Physicians, Indianapolis, IN, USA

Hal Douglas Kipfer Department of Radiology, Indiana Radiology Partners, Indianapolis, IN, USA

Jill Kremer IU Simon Cancer Center, Indiana University School of Medicine, Indianapolis, IN, USA

Kandice K. Ludwig Department of Surgery, Indiana University School of Medicine, Indianapolis, IN, USA

Sheila Mamandur Hiler Resident Physician, Indiana University School of Medicine, Indianapolis, IN, USA

Lida A. Mina Director of the Catherine Peachy Breast Cancer Prevention Program, Assistant Professor of Clinical Medicine. IU Simon Cancer Center, Indiana University School of Medicine, Indianapolis, IN, USA

Alain Mina Resident Physician, Kansas University Medical Center, Kansas City, KS, USA

Anna Maria Storniolo IU Simon Cancer Center, Indiana University School of Medicine, Indianapolis, IN, USA

Chapter 1
Introduction

Alain Mina and Lida A. Mina

1.1 Breast Cancer: The Magnitude of the Problem

Breast cancer is the most commonly diagnosed cancer and the number one cause of cancer-related deaths among women with 23 % of cancer diagnoses and 14 % of cancer deaths attributable to it [1]. A once feared and puzzling foe, its high prevalence and visibility to the naked eye lead to a historic interest and continuous rise in the knowledge and understanding of its facets [2]. Ancient Egyptian papyri were the first to describe the disease more than 3000 years ago and labeled it as "untreatable" [2]. From an imbalance in body fluids, referred to as the humoralism theory in the seventeenth century [3], to divine punishment [4], it was only until notable advances in surgical practices came to life in the nineteenth century that many of the disease's questions were answered. Not only did surgical advances elucidate the nature of the disease, but with the development of anesthesia and aseptic techniques in the second half of the nineteenth century, Dr. William Halsted perfected radical mastectomies, and the 20-year survival rates that were once 10 % plummeted to more than 50 % [3, 5], and the fate that once accompanied breast cancer diagnosis was no longer as dim. This "untreatable" entity with all its social implications is currently defined as a disease with early-local and late-systemic manifestations. Early detection and aggressive local and systemic therapy can be potentially curative.

A. Mina, MD
Resident Physician, Kansas University Medical Center, Kansas City, KS, USA

L.A. Mina, MD (✉)
Director of the Catherine Peachy Breast Cancer Prevention Program,
Assistant Professor of Clinical Medicine, IU Simon Cancer Center,
Indiana University School of Medicine, Indianapolis, IN, USA
e-mail: lmina@iu.edu

© Springer International Publishing Switzerland 2016
L.A. Mina et al. (eds.), *Breast Cancer Prevention and Treatment*,
DOI 10.1007/978-3-319-19437-0_1

1.2 Early Detection

The oldest version of "early" detection was and still is self-breast exam. A lot of controversy has surrounded breast self-exam, and the benefit of self-exam is still debatable. If one cruises the web, most renowned associations have specific recommendations and multistep processes on how to examine your own breast like the Susan G. Komen, the American Cancer Society, National Breast Cancer Foundation, and even Wikipedia, among other sites. Unfortunately, although it is a common practice, teaching breast self-examination does not seem to reduce breast cancer mortality and can increase false-positive rates that can lead to unnecessary imaging and biopsy procedures. Two large randomized trials, one in China involving more than 266,000 women and the other in Russia involving more than 120,300 women, did not demonstrate any mortality benefit from teaching breast self-examination [6, 7]. Another review looking at breast self-exam did not show any benefit for the rate of breast cancer diagnosis, the tumor size, stage, or even the death rate secondary to breast cancer [8]. Based on the above studies, the trend has shifted from recommending "breast self-examinations" to recommending "breast awareness." Organizations now encourage women 20 years and older to be aware of the normal appearance and feel their breasts, without using any systematic examination technique. The goal of breast self-awareness is for women to report any changes in their breasts to their primary care doctor [9–12]. Although there are no studies that prove the benefit of breast self-awareness, the number of times a woman finds a lump that turns out malignant warrants educating them to recognize changes or abnormalities in the breast. In summary, "Know your breast" is really what matters.

Clinical breast exam (CBE), although part of every gynecologist's and primary care doctor's exam, seems also to lack solid data. In a large review of controlled trials and case-control studies of CBE as a screening modality, CBE sensitivity and specificity were estimated to be 54 and 94 %, respectively [13]. Another study found that the addition of CBE to mammography increased mammography's sensitivity however with a higher false-positive rate [14]. The US Preventive Services Task Force (USPTF) questions the effectiveness of CBE because of the lack of well-designed large trials [15].

However, despite its shortcomings, we do believe that clinical breast exam should be part of the yearly physical exam of each individual woman.

The best screening modality to date remains mammography. Screening mammography was shown to decrease the rates of breast cancer mortality significantly. In a large meta-analysis of 13 randomized trials, screening mammography was shown to reduce the breast cancer-related mortality in women ages 50–74 years of age [16, 17].

1.3 Management

Management of breast cancer has come a long way. It started more than 100 years ago with a crude surgical approach and has evolved in recent years to a multidisciplinary approach involving surgical oncology, radiation oncology, and medical oncology, which has been associated with a significant decrease in breast cancer mortality. Our understanding of the biology of the disease and the intricacies of the heterogeneity of breast cancer has pushed targeted therapy in this area to new levels and opened the door for cure.

And though the golden era of treatment modalities is still ongoing, advances in early detection are on the rise as well, promising a brighter future for the breast cancer patient population and outstanding advances in early detection. But breast cancer remains the number one diagnosed cancer and the leading cause of cancer death in women worldwide. The only way to eradicate the disease would be to prevent it from happening in the first place.

1.4 Prevention

The only thing that beats cure remains prevention. Finding one less cancer means one life saved, whereas finding cancer even in the earliest of its stages can still claim one's life.

It was only recently that cancer was recognized as the outcome of interaction between environmental factors and genetic susceptibility. This modern definition of neoplastic disease opens the door to a newer more holistic approach to prevention: that of stratification of patients into groups of varying risk factors. Individualization of management is no longer limited to treatment but rather to prevention as well and is largely dictated by the risk factor group under which the patient falls. More than half of breast cancer diagnoses can be potentially claimed by well-established risk factors such as age, gender, race, weight, menopausal status, inherited genetic mutations, etc. Defining those factors and understanding the interplay between nature and nurture in this disease is the only way to prevent it from happening.

In the upcoming chapters, we will study and define those risk factors and lay out a plan of prevention in women especially at elevated risk for the disease.

References

1. Jemal A, Bray F, Center MM, Ferlay J, Ward E, Forman D. Global cancer statistics. Cancer J Clin. 2011;61(2):69.
2. Retief FP, Cilliers L. Breast cancer in antiquity. S Afr Med J. 2011;101(8):513–5.
3. A tumour through time. Will Tauxe. Nature 2015;527, S102-S103.
4. Yalom M. A history of the breast. New York: Alfred A Knopf; 1997. p. 234.
5. The results of operations for teh care of cancer of teh breast performed at the Johns Hopkins Hospital from June 1889 to January 1894. Ann Surg 1894;20:497.
6. Thomas DB, Gao DL, Ray RM, et al. Randomized trial of breast self-examination in Shanghai: final results. J Natl Cancer Inst. 2002;94(19):1445–57.
7. Semiglazov VF, Moiseyenko VM, Bavli JL, et al. The role of breast self-examination in early breast cancer detection (results of the 5-years USSR/WHO randomized study in Leningrad). Eur J Epidemiol. 1992;8(4):498–502.

8. Baxter N, Canadian Task Force on Preventive Health Care. Preventive health care, 2001 update: should women be routinely taught breast self-examination to screen for breast cancer? CMAJ. 2001;164(13):1837–46.

9. McCready T, Littlewood D, Jenkinson J. Breast self-examination and breast awareness: a literature review. J Clin Nurs. 2005;14(5):570–8.

10. National Comprehensive Cancer Network. NCCN clinical practice guidelines in oncology. Breast cancer screening and diagnosis, version 1.2011. http://www.nccn.org/professionals/physician_gls/pdf/breast-screening.pdf. [Registration required] Accessed 14 July 2012.

11. American College of Obstetricians-Gynecologists. Practice bulletin no. 122: breast cancer screening. Obstet Gynecol. 2011;118(2 pt 1):372–82.

12. Smith RA, Cokkinides V, Brawley OW. Cancer screening in the United States, 2009: a review of current American Cancer Society guidelines and issues in cancer screening. CA Cancer J Clin. 2009;59(1):27–41.

13. Barton MB, Harris R, Fletcher SW. The rational clinical examination. Does this patient have breast cancer? The screening clinical breast examination: should it be done? How? JAMA. 1999;282(13):1270–80.

14. Chiarelli AM, Majpruz V, Brown P, et al. The contribution of clinical breast examination to the accuracy of breast screening. J Natl Cancer Inst. 2009;101(18):1236–43.

15. Nelson HD, Tyne K, Naik A, et al. Screening for breast cancer: an update for the U.S. Preventive Services Task Force. Ann Intern Med. 2009;151(10):727–37.

16. Kerlikowske K. Efficacy of screening mammography among women aged 40 to 49 years and 50 to 69 years: comparison of relative and absolute benefit. J Natl Cancer Inst Monogr. 1997;22:79–86.

17. Nyström L, Andersson I, Bjurstam N, et al. Long-term effects of mammography screening: updated overview of the Swedish randomised trials [published correction appears in Lancet. 2002;360(9334):724]. Lancet. 2002;359(9310):909–19.

Chapter 2
Breast Cancer Risk Factors

Sheila Mamandur Hiler, Alain Mina, and Lida A. Mina

Breast cancer is the most common form of cancer among women and is the second most common cause of cancer-related mortality [1]. It is estimated that the number of new cases in 2014 is 232,670. A woman living in the USA has a one in eight lifetime risk of being diagnosed with breast cancer [2]. During the 1970s, this risk was 1 in 11. This increased risk can be attributed to changes in reproductive patterns, hormone therapy, obesity, lifestyle habits, and better detection [2]. Accordingly, it is important to identify those at increased risk, so that improved surveillance and risk-reducing interventions can be taken. This chapter will identify risk factors for breast cancer (Table 2.1).

2.1 Age

Age remains the number one independent risk factor associated with breast cancer [3]. Aging is an irreversible necessity that we can do nothing about. Aging cells in all of our organs and specifically in the breast tissue lose some of their ability to repair DNA malfunction. The buildup of DNA errors can lead to malignancy.

Chances of acquiring breast cancer increase with increasing age from a 5-year risk of 0.3 % at age 35 to 0.6 % at age 40, 1.8 % at age 60, and 2.0 % at age 80 [4]. The majority of new diagnosis of breast cancer (79 %) as well as related deaths

S.M. Hiler, MD, MS
Resident Physician, Indiana University School of Medicine, Indianapolis, IN, USA

A. Mina, MD
Resident Physician, Kansas University Medical Center, Kansas City, KS, USA

L.A. Mina, MD (✉)
Director of the Catherine Peachy Breast Cancer Prevention Program,
Assistant Professor of Clinical Medicine, IU Simon Cancer Center,
Indiana University School of Medicine, Indianapolis, IN, USA
e-mail: lmina@iu.edu

© Springer International Publishing Switzerland 2016
L.A. Mina et al. (eds.), *Breast Cancer Prevention and Treatment*,
DOI 10.1007/978-3-319-19437-0_2

Table 2.1 Breast cancer risk factors

Risk factor	*Effect on breast cancer risk*
Age	Increased age increases risk
Gender	Females are at higher risk
Race	Caucasian race is at higher risk
Endogenous estrogen related to reproductive factors	Earlier menarche and late menopause (usually)
Parity	Nulliparous women are at higher risk
Family history	Increased risk
Breast density	Higher density has higher risk
Transgenders	No increased risk
Radiation exposure	Increased risk in patients with BRCA mutations with radiation exposure before age 30 and with patients who have a history of mantle radiation
Fertility drugs	No association with risk

(88 %) occurs in women above the age of 50. And so increasing age is highly associated with the occurrence of breast cancer.

2.2   Gender

Another high risk for breast malignancies is gender. Women are 100 times more likely to be diagnosed with breast cancer than men. In the USA, 200,000 women are diagnosed with a breast malignancy annually as compared to 2000 cases in men [5]. In other words, the incidence of male breast cancer is less than 1 % compared to female breast cancer risk. The lifetime risk of male breast cancer is 1 in 1000. Males also tend to have breast cancer 5 years later than women, usually in the seventh decade of life. Recent trends have shown increases in the incidence of male breast cancer. Evidence from the SEER database shows that the incidence of male breast cancer over a 25-year period has increased from 0.86 to 1.08 per 100,000 population. This incidence rate is higher in black men than white men (reverse of females). This increased incidence may be due to better detection; however, obesity is also thought to play a role in this [6]. Because of its rarity, male breast cancer is understudied. The majority of diagnostic and management decisions are extrapolated from studies on female breast cancer [7]. Advancing age, radiation exposure, positive family history, and testicular abnormalities are associated with an increased risk of breast cancer in males. Estrogen exposure is also related to risk in males, and conditions such as obesity, chronic liver disease, and hyperlipidemia can be associated with male breast cancer. Unlike women, where only 1 % of breast cancer is associated with the BRCA gene mutations, 5–10 % of male breast cancer is associated with this [8].

2.3   Race

Another well-established risk for breast cancer occurrence is race. Population data from the Surveillance, Epidemiology, and End Results (SEER) database and the National Program of Cancer Registries showed a higher rate of breast cancer diagnoses in white women when compared to black women. It has been demonstrated that Caucasian race is an independent risk factor for breast cancer [9]. Rates in Caucasian women are 121.7 per 100,000 vs. 114.7 per 100,000 in African American women [9]. African Americans tended to present at a younger age, with a median age of 54 years vs. 61 years in Caucasian women. SEER data show that the incidence rate between 30 and 39 years is 48.36/100,000 in AA's vs. 40.79/100,000 in Caucasians. They tend to present with more locally advanced disease and had a greater breast cancer-specific mortality rate [10, 11]. These differences were initially largely attributed to lifestyle variations among the races as well as socioeconomic stressors (SES) or factors. However, the data on this is conflicting. Some studies have shown similar outcomes when adjusted for SES and equal access to healthcare; others have found that low SES and not race accounts for worse outcomes, and some studies have shown some racial disparity even after adjusted for SES [12].

Furthermore, we now know that the main driver is biology of the disease in African American women. African American women are more often to present with higher-grade tumors that have higher mitotic index, more tumor necrosis, and are poorly differentiated: the triple-negative tumors. Triple-negative tumors are usually larger, more advanced, and more likely to metastasize to axillary lymph nodes [4]. Those tumors tend to have more p53 mutations, higher mitotic index, more nuclear pleomorphism, and higher grade [4].

In summary, women less than 40 tend to present with worst histology (triple-negative disease) at a more advanced stage and are definitely more likely to be African American than Caucasians [11].

2.4   Estrogen and Other Hormones

Reproductive factors such as age at menarche, age at menopause, parity, infertility, and age at first pregnancy are widely accepted as highly significant risk factors for the development of breast cancer. The influence of these factors largely stems from their implications on extent of estrogen exposure. The longer and more significant this exposure is, the more likely it is to be associated with an increased risk of breast cancer. A younger age at menarche as well as an older age at menopause implies a more prolonged period of estrogen exposure and an increased rate of tissue growth, atypia, and subsequent tumor development.

Recent studies have shown that breast cancer risk increases with earlier menarche by a factor of 1.05 and with later menopause by a factor of 1.029 [13]. Women who had their first menstrual period before age 11 have in fact an RR 0.66 compared to those after age [14]. On the other hand, women who have their first live birth at age 30 or older have also an elevated risk of breast cancer [15]. Interestingly, however, these risks vary according to menopausal status. Age at menarche seems to only affect premenopausal risk. Age of first full-term pregnancy affects risk with both pre- and postmenopausal women [14].

And though multiparity's effect on breast cancer is a bit complex, nulliparity has been associated with a significantly increased risk of breast cancer, to the degree that it was labeled nuns' disease [16]. The "mystery of nuns' disease" was first brought to light in the fourteenth century when rates of breast cancer were dramatically elevated among nuns when compared to other groups of medieval women. It is assumed that the estrogen-suppressing/protective effects of childbearing and breastfeeding were lacking among this population and manifested in much higher rates of disease [17].

Studies have also focused quite a bit on the effects of endogenous estrogen on precancerous lesions like ductal carcinoma in situ (DCIS). Factors specifically linked to ductal carcinoma in situ include later age at menopause and later age of first pregnancy [15]. Women who have menopause at age 55 years or older have 39 % increased risk of DCIS compared to women who have menopause between ages 45 and 54 [15].

Another somewhat worrisome exposure with regard to cancer development is hormone replacement therapy (HRT). HRT has been the subject of great controversy and concern among patients. Studies have demonstrated a clear increase in breast cancer rates with menopausal hormone therapy; however, the risk differs whether be it with unopposed estrogen or combined estrogen-progestin therapies. In the placebo-controlled Women's Health Initiative (WHI) study, the combined estrogen-progestin arm had a significant increase in risk of developing breast cancer at an average follow-up of 5.6 years [18]. But when looking at the arm with unopposed estrogen, the risk of breast cancer did not seem to be increased at all which was really surprising [19]. This is currently still a matter of controversy and we shall be discussing that risk factor further in a later chapter.

Further support of the estrogen role in breast cancer risk is the standard use of estrogen blockers or modulators in post- and premenopausal women as a very successful means to decreasing breast cancer risk. Both tamoxifen and raloxifene are selective estrogen receptor modulators (SERMs) used for the treatment of breast cancer. SERMs have estrogen agonist activity in some tissues, and antagonist activity in other tissues such as the breast, and can reduce the risk of breast cancer [20]. Tamoxifen used prophylactically in high-risk women has been shown to reduce the risk of breast cancer by 1/3, although risks and benefits must be considered [21]. Letrozole, an aromatase inhibitor, which prevents estrogen synthesis, is also used in the treatment of breast cancer and has been shown to improve disease-free survival [22].

2.5   Transgender and Breast Cancer Risk

There has recently been an interest in the media on transgender persons. Many patients with gender dysphoria are treated with cross-sex hormones. The use of this exogenous hormone raises the question of whether there is an increased risk of breast cancer. One large cohort study done through the Veterans Administration

(VA) found that transgender patients on cross-sex hormones (CSH) did not have an increased risk of breast cancer in either sex, as compared to the general population. Supporting this evidence is the fact that exposure to estrogen and antiandrogens during treatment of prostate cancer has no increased risk of breast cancer, despite having the known side effect of gynecomastia [3]. Another study also evaluated transgender persons, with male to female patients on estrogen and androgen deprivation medications and female to male patients on testosterone. This study also found no increased risk with cross-sex hormone treatment. The incidence of breast cancer in both groups was similar to risk of male breast cancer [23].

2.6   Radiation

Radiation exposure is also a risk for breast cancer, particularly in patients who had received mantle radiotherapy after a diagnosis of Hodgkin's lymphoma. In those patients, the risk of breast cancer is inversely related to age of treatment [24]. Patients diagnosed at a younger age have a significantly higher risk. Patients that have either the BRCA1/2 mutation are at increased risk of breast cancer with any exposure to diagnostic radiation before the age of 30. Specifically, increased number of radiographs before age 30 does correlate with an increased risk of breast cancer. Mammography before age 30 is also associated with increased risk. There is no evidence that radiation exposure after age 30 has an increased risk [25]. There is no association between mammography and increased risk of breast cancer. Also, the risk of breast cancer associated with radiation decreases with increasing age at exposure. Risk is not observed until 10–15 years after exposure [26].

2.7   Fertility Drugs

A woman's reproductive history is a known risk factor for breast cancer; however, approximately 9 % of couples have some form of infertility and 56 % of couples seek treatment for infertility. Many of these fertility treatments are hormonal based. This raises the question of whether fertility agents increase breast cancer risk [27].

Clomiphene citrate, a fertility agent used to stimulate ovulation, has no associated increased risk of breast cancer and no relationship between the number of cycles and breast cancer risk. In fact, there may be a lower risk of breast cancer with increased number of clomiphene cycles [27]. There is no association between IVF and risk of breast cancer. Letrozole, an aromatase inhibitor, is used as a fertility agent in patients with endometriosis, PCOS, and unexplained fertility. There is no increased risk between letrozole/aromatase inhibitors and breast cancer. Overall, there is no association between fertility drugs and breast cancer risk, and in fact there may be a protective role of ovarian stimulation [28].

References

1. Siegel RL, Miller KD, Jemal A. Cancer statistics, 2015. CA Cancer J Clin. 2015;65(1):5–29.
2. American Cancer Society. Breast Cancer Facts and Figures 2015–2016: Atlanta: American Cancer Society, Inc. 2015.
3. Hartz AJ, He T. Cohort study of risk factors for breast cancer in post menopausal women. Epidemiol Health. 2013;35:e2013003.
4. Breast Cancer Risk Assessment Tool. National Institutes of Health. Available at: www.cancer.gov/bcrisktool.
5. Jemal A, Bray F, Center MM, et al. Global cancer statistics. CA Cancer J Clin. 2011;61:69.
6. Humphries MP, Jordan VC, Speirs V. Obesity and male breast cancer: provocative parallels? BMC Med. 2015;13:134.
7. Korde LA. Male breast cancer: a Study in Small Steps. Oncologist. 2015;20(6):584–5.
8. Brown GR, Jones KT. Incidence of breast cancer in a cohort of 5,135 transgender veterans. Breast Cancer Res Treat. 2015;149(1):191–8.
9. Danforth Jr DN. Disparities in breast cancer outcomes between Caucasian and African American women: a model for describing the relationship of biological and nonbiological factors. Breast Cancer Res. 2013;15(3):208.
10. CDC. Vital signs: racial disparities in breast cancer severity — United States, 2005–2009. MMWR Morb Mortal Wkly Rep. 2012;61:922.
11. Carey LA, Perou CM, Livasy CA, et al. Race, breast cancer subtypes, and survival in the Carolina Breast Cancer Study. JAMA. 2006;295:2492.
12. Parise CA, Caggiano V. Disparities in race/ethnicity and socioeconomic status: risk of mortality of breast cancer patients in the California Cancer Registry, 2000–2010. BMC Cancer. 2013;13:449.
13. Collaborative Group on Hormonal Factors in Breast Cancer. Menarche, menopause, and breast cancer risk: individual participant meta-analysis, including 118 964 women with breast cancer from 117 epidemiological studies. Lancet Oncol. 2012;13(11):1141–51.
14. Clavel-Chapelon F. Differential effects of reproductive factors on the risk of pre- and postmenopausal breast cancer. Results from a large cohort of French women. Br J Cancer. 2002;86(5):723–7.
15. Kabat GC, et al. Reproductive and menstrual factors and risk of ductal carcinoma in situ of the breast in a cohort of postmenopausal women. Cancer Causes Control. 2011;22(10):1415–24.
16. Gleicher N. Why are reproductive cancers more common in nulliparous women? Reprod Biomed Online. 2013;26(5):416–19.
17. Bruzzi P, Negri E, La Vecchia C, et al. Short term increase in risk of breast cancer after full term pregnancy. BMJ. 1988;297:1096.
18. Rossouw JE, Anderson GL, Prentice RL, et al. Risks and benefits of estrogen plus progestin in healthy postmenopausal women: principal results. From the Women's Health Initiative randomized controlled trial. JAMA. 2002;288(3):321.
19. Prentice RL, Chlebowski RT, Stefanick ML, et al. Conjugated equine estrogens and breast cancer risk in the Women's Health Initiative clinical trial and observational study. Am J Epidemiol. 2008;167(12):1407.
20. Vogel VG. The NSABP Study of Tamoxifen and Raloxifene (STAR) trial. Expert Rev Anticancer Ther. 2009;9(1):51–60.
21. Cuzick J, et al. First results from the International Breast Cancer Intervention Study (IBIS-I): a randomised prevention trial. Lancet. 2002;360(9336):817–24.
22. Goss PE. Letrozole in the extended adjuvant setting: MA.17. Breast Cancer Res Treat. 2007;105 Suppl 1:45–53.
23. Gooren LJ, et al. Breast cancer development in transsexual subjects receiving cross-sex hormone treatment. J Sex Med. 2013;10(12):3129–34.
24. Basu SK, Schwartz C, Fisher SG, et al. Unilateral and bilateral breast cancer in women surviving pediatric Hodgkin's disease. Int J Radiat Oncol Biol Phys. 2008;72(1):34.

25. Pijpe A, et al. Exposure to diagnostic radiation and risk of breast cancer among carriers of BRCA1/2 mutations: retrospective cohort study (GENE-RAD-RISK). BMJ. 2012;345:e5660.
26. Andrieu N, et al. Effect of chest X-rays on the risk of breast cancer among BRCA1/2 mutation carriers in the international BRCA1/2 carrier cohort study: a report from the EMBRACE, GENEPSO, GEO-HEBON, and IBCCS Collaborators' Group. J Clin Oncol. 2006; 24(21):3361–6.
27. Zreik TG, et al. Fertility drugs and the risk of breast cancer: a meta-analysis and review. Breast Cancer Res Treat. 2010;124(1):13–26.
28. Tomao F, et al. Clinical use of fertility agents and risk of breast cancer: a recent update for an old problem. Curr Opin Obstet Gynecol. 2014;26(3):130–7.

Chapter 3
Lifestyle and Breast Cancer

Sheila Mamandur Hiler and Lida A. Mina

Risk factors for breast cancer were addressed in Chap. 2; however, this can only explain about 40 % of all breast cancer cases [1]. It is known that lifestyle factors can influence the risk of breast cancer. 90 % of cancers are linked to environmental exposure so one strategy for controlling the rates of breast cancer would be through prevention. The fact that incidence rates differ between western and eastern countries also suggests an important role for environmental factors [1].

This chapter will address those factors and how they can be implemented into cancer prevention approaches. The American Cancer Society has released guidelines for lifestyle measures which can prevent breast cancer [2].

3.1 Exercise

There have been multiple studies demonstrating that physical activity can lower risk of breast cancer by 10–20 % compared to those who are inactive. This benefit may be due to the effect on BMI, hormones, or energy balance [2]. It is thought that physical inactivity is responsible for 10 % of breast cancer. One study demonstrated that a 25 % decrease in inactivity may reduce 1.3 million deaths annually. However, findings from studies have been variable and this is thought to be due to variability in measures of physical activity [1].

S.M. Hiler, MD, MS
Resident Physician, Indiana University School of Medicine, Indianapolis, IN, USA

L.A. Mina, MD (✉)
Director of the Catherine Peachy Breast Cancer Prevention Program,
Assistant Professor of Clinical Medicine, IU Simon Cancer Center,
Indiana University School of Medicine, Indianapolis, IN, USA
e-mail: lmina@iu.edu

© Springer International Publishing Switzerland 2016
L.A. Mina et al. (eds.), *Breast Cancer Prevention and Treatment*,
DOI 10.1007/978-3-319-19437-0_3

Borch et al. demonstrated that in women who have a low physical activity level at age 30, there is an increased risk of ER+/PR+ breast tumors [3]. It is thought that the association between physical activity and breast cancer risk is mediated through molecular pathways, specifically, exercise can decrease breast cancer risk by causing weight loss as well as possibly decreasing concentration of sex hormones, insulin-like growth factor 1, sex hormone binding globulin as well as modulating inflammation [1]. Activation of the insulin growth factor receptor by IGFs results in autophosphorylation and activation of intrinsic tyrosine kinase which then results in proliferation and differentiation, leading to cancer [4].

Physical activity also affects other risk factors such as obesity and insulin resistance [5]. Obesity and overweight are known to increase risk of breast cancer. A study involving 1000 women with breast cancer found that 30 % were obese and another 32 % were overweight. Furthermore, the incidence of metabolic syndrome is estimated to be 50 % in patients with breast cancer and obesity is associated with worse prognosis [4]. In postmenopausal women, increased weight is associated with increased risk; however, this association is not found in premenopausal women (obesity may actually be protective in this population), suggesting a role for hormones. Also, weight gain during middle adulthood confers increased risk of breast cancer [5]. Adipose tissue contains high levels of aromatase, which convert androgens to estrogens, leading to increased breast cancer risk [6].

3.2   Obesity

Obesity and metabolic syndrome are influenced by diet, which has also been shown to affect the risk of breast cancer and can explain part of the difference in incidence rates between western and eastern countries. Western developed countries have a diet high in animal products, fat, and sugar. Fat intake is associated with an increased risk of breast cancer; however, interventions to reduce fat intake have shown no decrease in the risk of breast cancer [5]. On the contrary, developing countries eat more starchy foods, with low consumption of animal products, fat, and sugar [1].

Diet plays a role in risk through chemical carcinogens in unhealthy foods versus high antioxidants in healthy foods. Multiple studies have demonstrated a significant difference between foods consumed by patients with breast cancer and those without, so diet modification plays a large role in breast cancer prevention.

Antioxidants can decrease cancer risk by promoting DNA repair and metabolic detoxification and decreasing estrogens.

Unhealthy diets can stimulate production of IGF-1 [1]. As described above, insulin-like growth factors activate cell proliferation, and higher concentrations of IGF-1 are associated with increased risk of breast cancer. It has been demonstrated that increased protein and dairy intake result in higher levels of IGF-1 [7]. Evidence also indicates that diets with a high glycemic index are associated with increased risk of breast cancer [8].

Evidence has shown that increased intake of fruits and vegetables, limiting caloric intake, and eating whole grains can prevent breast cancer. Eating vegetables

Table 3.1 Lifestyle changes and breast cancer risk

Lifestyle factors	Affect on breast cancer risk
Physical activity	Decreased
Obesity/overweight	Increased risk
Diet	High fat – increased risk
	Mediterranean diet – decreased risk
Alcohol intake	Increased risk
Caffeine	Conflicting data, but overall seems to have decreased risk
Soy intake	Decreased
Hormone replacement therapy and OCPs	Increased risk
Vitamin D deficiency	Increased risk
Herbal supplements	No association

decreases breast cancer risk by 6 % and eating fruits is associated with a 12 % decrease. It has also been demonstrated that there is an inverse relationship between use of oils with high polyunsaturated fats (such as olive oil) and breast cancer [9].

Ataoillahl et al. confirmed that there is a significant relationship between breast cancer and unhealthy nutritional choices as indicated in Table 3.1. They showed a significant difference both in the food groups and in types of food consumed by patients with and without breast cancer. They also found a higher consumption of fruits and vegetables in healthy people compared to those with cancer. This can be explained by the fact that intake of vitamin B6, B12, and folate is associated with lower risk of breast cancer, and these are found in fruits and vegetables [9].

Data suggests that following a Mediterranean diet can lead to a decreased risk of breast cancer. Hallmarks of a Mediterranean diet include olive oil, cereals, fresh or dried fruits and vegetables, fish, dairy, and meat; however, cereals, fruits, and vegetables seem to have the most benefit. There is an inverse association with the likelihood of breast cancer and adherence to a Mediterranean diet, particularly in women of normal weight and postmenopausal women [10]. This associated reduction in breast cancer risk is also stronger in receptor-negative tumors [11].

3.3 Alcohol

Alcohol intake is another risk factor for breast cancer. Alcohol disrupts the metabolism and absorption of folate. It also increases estrogen levels by impairing metabolism. Ethanol is also thought to increase risk through formation of reactive oxygen species, which in turn causes DNA damage and chromosomal abnormalities. Furthermore, it can induce cell proliferation and expression of ER/PR receptors [1].

Alcohol intake has also been strongly linked to increased risk of ER+ tumors. As demonstrated earlier, the American Cancer Society recommends no more than one alcoholic drink per day for women and no more than two drinks per day for men [2].

Studies have shown an increased risk of 7–12 % for each drink of alcohol consumed per day. This risk appears to be dose-dependent and does not depend upon the type of alcohol consumed. Smith-Warner et al. demonstrated that alcohol consumption is associated with a linear increase in breast cancer risk [12].

Some studies have reported alcohol-related risk could be attenuated by consumption of folic acid; however, more evidence is needed to support this. Also, in contrast to tobacco use, alcohol intake does not change survival after diagnosis [5]. In postmenopausal women, the risk is doubled in those consuming more than two drinks weekly. Also, the degree of risk varies with age of first drink, menopausal status, amount of ingested alcohol, and polymorphisms of an individual's genes [1].

3.4 Caffeine

The role of caffeine on the risk of breast cancer is unclear. Some studies have linked coffee consumption to benign breast disease, which can then lead to breast cancer; however, other studies have suggested a possible benefit [13]. Ganmaa et al. conducted a large cohort study and found a significant inverse association of caffeine intake with breast cancer, which was stronger in postmenopausal women than premenopausal women [14]. Also, a meta-analysis published by Tang et al. found an association between coffee intake and decreased risk of breast cancer in the USA and Europe [13]. Another meta-analysis done [15] showed a negative association of coffee/caffeine intake with breast cancer across multiple subgroups including country of study, BMI, and ER and PR status. This association was significant in postmenopausal women but not premenopausal women. They also found a dose-response, linear relationship between coffee intake and breast cancer risk, with a 2 % reduction in risk with every two cups/day increase in coffee consumption.

There have been multiple mechanisms proposed to explain the reduced risk of breast cancer associated with caffeine intake. The major components of coffee, caffeic acid, and caffeine have been shown to inhibit DNA methylation in breast cancer cells. Coffee intake is also inversely associated with circulating levels of inflammatory markers and insulin resistance, which play a role in breast cancer. Also, coffee may decrease risk by influencing estrogen metabolism [16].

3.5 Soy

Soy intake is also thought to contribute to breast cancer risk and has been suggested to explain the lower incidence of breast cancer in Asian countries, where soy intake in high. A meta-analysis done by Trock et al. showed that high soy intake was associated with reduced breast cancer risk. In ten of the studies they used, the inverse relationship was stronger in premenopausal women. Soybeans contain the isoflavones genistein and daidzein. It is thought that these isoflavones compete with estrogen receptors, and they may have antiproliferative, anti-angiogenic, anti-oxidative, and anti-inflammatory properties [17]. Also, genistein can induce mammary cell differentiation and activates ER-β, a protein with apoptotic activity. Daidzein has been found to increase tamoxifen efficacy at physiologic levels in rat models [17].

Wu et al. also conducted a meta-analysis which showed similar results. They found that in Asians, there was a decreased risk of breast cancer with increasing soy intake. Compared to the lowest dose of soy food intake (<5 mg isoflavones/day), there was intermediate risk with 10 mg and lowest risk in those with high soy intake (>20 mg isoflavones/day). However, this association was not found in Western populations, which is thought to be related to overall low soy intake [18].

3.6   Exogenous Hormone

Hormone replacement therapy is also associated with breast cancer risk, specifically with increased risk. Oral contraceptives (OCs) are thought to increase risk of breast cancer by 10–30 % [2]. Risk is highest when OCs are used during teenage years, but risk returns to normal after stopping OCs for 10 years or more [6]. However, most studies have only looked at high-dose estrogen OCs, so risk associated with the low-dose forms is not clear. Recent studies provide no evidence that current use of OCs increase breast cancer risk, which is likely due to the fact that OCs today contain less estrogen and progestin than previous decades [6].

The most well-known study looking at hormone replacement was the Women's Health Initiative (WHI). They found a 24 % increased risk of invasive breast cancer with estrogen plus progesterone therapy compared to placebo. This risk was most evident in the third year of use for previous HRT users versus the fourth year of use for never users. Also, estrogen plus progesterone therapy (EPT) was associated with more abnormal mammograms, and increased breast density, which as discussed in Chap. 2, is associated with increased breast cancer risk. The WHI also found that breast cancer risk decreased rapidly after discontinuation.

Conversely, the WHI found no increased risk of breast cancer in the estrogen therapy (ET) group alone; however, it is important to note that this was less than 5 years of unopposed estrogen exposure and may be different with longer exposure. Estrogen therapy alone also increased mammographic density but to a lesser extent than EPT. Also, in women who developed breast cancer on HRT, the tumor size, histology, and HER2 status were similar compared to those on placebo. However, those on EPT had a higher risk of being node-positive and had a higher risk of mortality compared to placebo [19].

If hormone replacement therapy is needed, then initial breast cancer risk should be considered. It is important to note that the effect of HT on breast cancer risk does not seem to be modified by the traditional breast cancer risk factors such as family history. However, some studies have suggested that it can modify risk associated with obesity, with increased risk in women with lower BMI. Regarding HRT in breast cancer survivors, there is evidence that it is associated with twice the risk of recurrence [19].

3.7 Vitamin D Deficiency

There is evidence that suggests vitamin D may have a protective role in breast cancer and thus deficiency can be a risk factor for breast cancer. Vitamin D is obtained through diet and synthesized in our body from sunlight exposure, with the majority of vitamin D coming from sunlight exposure [20]. There is evidence of an inverse relationship between sunlight exposure and breast cancer incidence and mortality [18]. High sunlight exposure can decrease breast cancer risk by 25–65 % in women who live in states with high solar radiation. This is thought to be due to higher vitamin D levels, supported by the fact that vitamin D levels are 13 % higher in women living in southern states [21]. Dietary vitamin D may also have a role in breast cancer risk. There may be a trend toward less breast cancer in women who consume greater than 400 IU/day of vitamin D [22].

3.8 Herbal Supplements

With the advent of alternative medicine, the use of supplements thought to have anti-inflammatory and anticancer properties has increased. Supplements used to treat menopausal symptoms, such as black cohosh, dong quai, soy, or St. John's wort, have no association with increased breast cancer risk. Fish oil is thought to decrease breast cancer risk. There is no association between breast cancer and anti-inflammatory supplements such as glucosamine and chondroitin [23].

Bibliography

1. Kruk J. Lifestyle components and primary breast cancer prevention. Asian Pac J Cancer Prev. 2014;15(24):10543–55.
2. American Cancer Society. Breast cancer facts & figures 2013–2014. Atlanta: American Cancer Society, Inc; 2013.
3. Borch KB, et al. Physical activity and the risk of postmenopausal breast cancer–the Norwegian Women and Cancer Study. J Negat Results Biomed. 2014;13:3.
4. Zielinska HA, et al. Epithelial-to-mesenchymal transition in breast cancer: a role for insulin-like growth factor I and insulin-like growth factor-binding protein 3? Breast Cancer (Dove Med Press). 2015;7:9–19.
5. Hashemi SH, Karimi S, Mahboobi H. Lifestyle changes for prevention of breast cancer. El Phys. 2014;6(3):894–905.
6. Hilakivi-Clarke L, de Assis S, Warri A. Exposures to synthetic estrogens at different times during the life, and their effect on breast cancer risk. J Mammary Gland Biol Neoplasia. 2013;18(1):25–42.

7. Bradbury KE, et al. The association of plasma IGF-I with dietary, lifestyle, anthropometric, and early life factors in postmenopausal women. Growth Horm IGF Res. 2015;25(2):90–5.
8. Mullie P, et al. Relation between breast cancer and high glycemic index or glycemic load: a meta-analysis of prospective cohort studies. Crit Rev Food Sci Nutr. 2015;56(1):152–9.
9. Ataollahi M, Sedighi S, Masoumi SZ. Nutritional and unhealthy behaviors in women with and without breast cancer. Iran Red Crescent Med J. 2014;16(9):e19684.
10. Mourouti N, et al. Adherence to the Mediterranean diet is associated with lower likelihood of breast cancer: a case-control study. Nutr Cancer. 2014;66(5):810–7.
11. Buckland G, et al. Adherence to the mediterranean diet and risk of breast cancer in the European prospective investigation into cancer and nutrition cohort study. Int J Cancer. 2013;132(12):2918–27.
12. Smith-Warner SA, et al. Alcohol and breast cancer in women: a pooled analysis of cohort studies. JAMA. 1998;279(7):535–40.
13. Tang N, et al. Coffee consumption and risk of breast cancer: a metaanalysis. Am J Obstet Gynecol. 2009;200(3):290.e1–9.
14. Ganmaa D, et al. Coffee, tea, caffeine and risk of breast cancer: a 22-year follow-up. Int J Cancer. 2008;122(9):2071–6.
15. Jiang W, Wu Y, Jiang X. Coffee and caffeine intake and breast cancer risk: an updated dose-response meta-analysis of 37 published studies. Gynecol Oncol. 2013;129(3):620–9.
16. Gierach GL, et al. Coffee intake and breast cancer risk in the NIH-AARP diet and health study cohort. Int J Cancer. 2012;131(2):452–60.
17. Wu AH, et al. Epidemiology of soy exposures and breast cancer risk. Br J Cancer. 2008;98(1):9–14.
18. Trock BJ, Hilakivi-Clarke L, Clarke R. Meta-analysis of soy intake and breast cancer risk. J Natl Cancer Inst. 2006;98(7):459–71.
19. Chen WY. Postmenopausal hormone therapy and breast cancer risk: current status and unanswered questions. Endocrinol Metab Clin North Am. 2011;40(3):509–18, viii.
20. Shao T, Klein P, Grossbard ML. Vitamin D and breast cancer. Oncologist. 2012;17(1):36–45.
21. John EM, et al. Vitamin D and breast cancer risk: the NHANES I Epidemiologic follow-up study, 1971–1975 to 1992. National Health and Nutrition Examination Survey. Cancer Epidemiol Biomarkers Prev. 1999;8(5):399–406.
22. Gissel T, et al. Intake of vitamin D and risk of breast cancer – a meta-analysis. J Steroid Biochem Mol Biol. 2008;111(3–5):195–9.
23. Brasky TM, et al. Specialty supplements and breast cancer risk in the VITamins And Lifestyle (VITAL) Cohort. Cancer Epidemiol Biomarkers Prev. 2010;19(7):1696–708.

Chapter 4
Genetic Evaluation and Testing

Cindy Hunter

The Surveillance, Epidemiology, and End Results of the National Cancer Institute (SEER) data indicate the general population risk for developing breast cancer in the United States is 1 in 8 or 12.3 % based on 2010–2012 data (http://seer.cancer.gov/statfacts/html/breast.html). The majority of breast cancers develop independent of highly penetrant germline (inherited) mutations, and in these cases, genetic evaluation and testing is not expected to be of significant clinical benefit. Given the relatively high frequency in the general population, it is also not unexpected for two or three sporadically occurring breast cancers to occur within an extended family. However, the presence of multiple diagnoses of breast cancer, especially if within first- and second-degree relatives and if earlier onset, should lead to consideration of genetic evaluation.

4.1   Genetic Evaluation

The primary purpose of a genetic evaluation is to assess the likelihood of the patient, or family, having an inherited condition predisposing to cancer and whether genetic testing for cancer susceptibility is medically indicated. Secondly, establishing the prior probability of a germline mutation being present is integral when interpreting the results of genetic testing, especially if no germline mutation or a genetic variant of unknown clinical significance were to be identified.

C. Hunter, MS, LCGC
Medical and Molecular Genetics Department, Indiana University Health Physicians,
Indianapolis, IN, USA
e-mail: chunter2@IUHealth.org

© Springer International Publishing Switzerland 2016   21
L.A. Mina et al. (eds.), *Breast Cancer Prevention and Treatment*,
DOI 10.1007/978-3-319-19437-0_4

Genetic evaluation includes the following components:

Three-Generation Pedigree Medical history information is gathered for the patient, the patient's children, siblings, nieces, nephews, parents, aunts, uncles, cousins, and grandparents, both maternal and paternal sides. Medical history information should include current age or age at death, any diagnoses of benign and malignant tumors, age at diagnosis and treatment, history of risk-reducing procedures (e.g., oophorectomy), environmental exposures, and whether any family member has undergone genetic testing for cancer susceptibility.

Documenting the Tumor Diagnoses Pathology information for the reported tumor/cancer diagnoses in family members is particularly important. This information documents the diagnosis and age at diagnosis which allows for more accurate assessment of the patient's risk for developing cancer and of the likelihood of an underlying genetic predisposition. Reports of ovarian cancer are commonly encountered when assessing a family history of breast cancer, but frequently, upon further inquiry, the patient learns the affected relative had some other type of tumor or issue. Schneider et al. reported an accuracy rate of 74 % for reports of ovarian cancer and that accuracy of reports significantly lessened for second-degree relatives (aunts, uncles, grandparents) in comparison to first-degree relatives (parents, siblings, children) [42]. Reports of male breast cancer have in some cases actually been skin cancer involving the skin of the breast or benign tumors involving the breast, e.g., lipoma (personal experience).

Tumor documentation also allows for more definitive assessment regarding the clinical utility of genetic testing. Associations exist between particular pathological findings and likelihood of certain mutations being identified. Triple-negative breast cancers are associated with a higher incidence of germline *BRCA1* mutations. Lobular breast cancers, in the context of a personal or family history of diffuse gastric cancer, are indicative of *CDH1* involvement. Serous borderline ovarian (low malignant potential) cancers and non-epithelial ovarian carcinomas are not component tumors of BRCA1/2-associated hereditary breast and ovarian cancer syndrome (HBOC).

Ancestry Likewise, ancestry may direct decisions regarding genetic testing. Certain population groups are associated with founder mutations, a specific gene mutation observed at a high frequency within a specific population. The most common example in the United States involves the Ashkenazi (Central/Eastern European) Jewish population. Individuals who are of Ashkenazi Jewish descent have a 2–3 % chance for carrying 1 of 3 *BRCA1/2* founder mutations (*BRCA1* 187delAG, *BRCA1* 5385insC, and *BRCA2* 6174delT). More than 95 % of Ashkenazi Jewish families with hereditary breast and ovarian cancer carry one of these three mutations. In these cases, genetic testing may focus on these three specific mutations which allows for more definitive results and at significantly less cost. Other populations with founder mutations include the Icelandic, Dutch, and Mexican populations; however, within the United States, genetic testing strategies are currently less impacted by this information.

4.2   Guidelines for Genetic Evaluation and/or Testing

Guidelines for when genetic evaluation by a genetics professional should be considered have been published. The National Comprehensive Cancer Network (NCCN, www.nccn.org) criteria are reviewed, revised, and published annually in NCCN Clinical Practice Guidelines in Oncology: Genetic/Familial High-Risk Assessment: Breast and Ovarian Cancer [30]. Criteria established by The American College of Medical Genetics and Genomics (ACMG) and National Society of Genetic Counselors are listed in Table 4.1 [16]. In cases of patients presenting for family history of breast cancer, if an affected first- or second-degree relative meets these criteria, exploration of whether that relative would consent to genetic evaluation would greatly benefit the patient's medical care.

Professional cancer and genetic societies recommend consultation with cancer genetic professionals for pre-and post-genetic testing assessment and counseling. Genetic counselors and medical geneticists are trained to elicit detailed and complete pedigrees while keeping the differential diagnoses in mind and are expert at explaining complex genetic information to patients including implications of a genetic diagnosis to them and their families.

Involvement of genetic health professions increases accuracy of genetic test ordering. The genetics division of ARUP, a national reference laboratory, published data in 2014 reporting on the involvement of genetic counselors in reviewing all orders for complex germline molecular testing. Approximately 26 % of all requests for complex molecular genetic tests were changed following genetic counselor review during the 21-month study period. Incorrect orders represented 61 % of the changes and included errors such as ordering full gene analysis when a gene panel was more appropriate or when the familial mutation was already known, ordering the wrong test, and duplicate

Table 4.1 ACMG/NSGC criteria warranting assessment for cancer predisposition [16]

Female breast cancer diagnosed at or before age 50
Triple-negative breast cancer diagnosed at or before 60
≥2 primary breast cancers in the same individual
Ashkenazi Jewish ancestry and breast cancer at any age
≥3 cases of breast, ovarian, pancreatic, and/or aggressive prostate cancer in close relatives, including the patient
Breast cancer and one additional Li–Fraumeni syndrome tumor (soft-tissue sarcoma, osteosarcoma, brain tumor, adrenocortical carcinoma, leukemia, bronchoalveolar carcinoma, colorectal cancer) in the same person or in two relatives, one diagnosed at or before age 45
Breast cancer and ≥1 Peutz–Jeghers polyp in the same person
Lobular breast cancer and diffuse gastric cancer in the same person
Lobular breast cancer in one relative and diffuse gastric cancer in another relative, one diagnosed before age 50
Breast cancer and ≥2 additional Cowden syndrome criteria (Table 4.4) in the same person
Male breast cancer

testing. The resulting cost savings were calculated to be $1.2 million [28]. A 2015 study also found that involvement of a genetic counselor or medical geneticist in *BRCA1/2* genetic testing reduced the frequency of incorrect orders by about half [7].

Online searchable databases are available for genetic counselors and medical geneticists: American Board of Medical Genetics and Genomics (www.acmg.org) and National Society of Genetic Counselors (www.nsgc.org).

4.3 "Familial" Versus "Hereditary" Cancer

About 5–10 % of breast cancer is due to a single highly penetrant germline mutation. Hereditary cancer is diagnosed when a lineage demonstrates certain characteristics (Table 4.2; Fig. 4.1). In patients presenting due to a family history of breast cancer, risk for carrying a germline mutation associated with hereditary breast cancer should be considered if they report an affected first- or second-degree relative and the following, within the same lineage:

- Multiple occurrences of early-onset breast cancer in successive generations (e.g., autosomal dominant pattern of cancer)
- ≥1 family member developing multiple primary breast cancers
- ≥1 family member developing both primary breast and primary epithelial ovarian cancer
- ≥1 occurrences of male breast cancer
- ≥2 occurrences of uncommon or rare cancers including soft-tissue sarcomas, osteosarcomas, diffuse gastric cancer, and pancreatic adenocarcinoma
- Ashkenazi Jewish ancestry

Hereditary forms of cancer follow autosomal dominant inheritance. Each child a mutation carrier has will have a 1-in-2 (50 %) chance to inherit the familial mutation.

About 10–20 % of breast cancer is "familial," resulting from a multifactorial predisposition. Familial cancer is characterized by a clustering of cancer within a lineage in the absence of characteristics of hereditary cancer (Fig. 4.1). There are often an absence of a clear-cut inheritance pattern and an absence of multiple primary tumors, and cancers are diagnosed in later middle ages (sixth and seventh

Table 4.2 Features indicative of hereditary cancer

Multiple occurrences of the same or related cancer in successive generations
Autosomal dominant pattern of cancer
Multiple early-onset diagnoses (diagnosed 50 years or younger)
≥2 occurrences of uncommon or rare cancers (i.e., male breast cancer, adrenocortical carcinoma pancreatic adenocarcinoma) within the same lineage
Development of ≥2 primary cancers in an individual

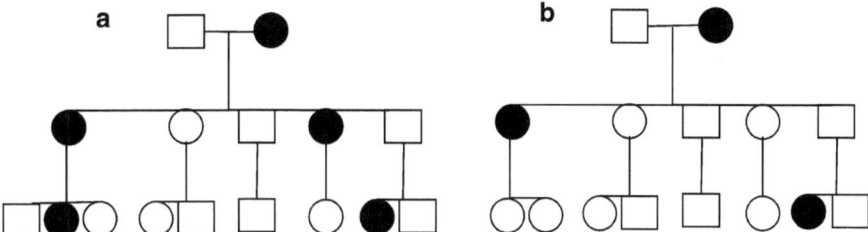

Fig. 4.1 (**a**) Autosomal dominant inheritance; (**b**) familial/multifactorial inheritance. Key: *circle* female, *square* male, *colored-in* diagnosed with breast cancer

decades). Familial predisposition derives from the joint effect of multiple factors including shared environmental risk factors, interaction of low/moderate penetrant genetic mutations, and interaction of genes and environment/lifestyle choices.

The characterization of familial breast cancer is evolving due the recent identification of moderate penetrant genes. These studies are demonstrating that, unlike highly penetrant genetic conditions, genotype is not the primary risk factor for developing breast cancer. As cases in point, *PALB2*- and *CHEK2*-associated breast cancer risk appears to be modified by strength of family history. Antoniou and colleagues published in 2014 the first large study of *PALB2* loss-of-function mutation carriers and found the breast cancer risk at age 50 to be approximately 33 % but increased to 58 % if there were two affected first-degree relatives [2]. A meta-analysis of the *CHEK2* 1100delC mutation in early-onset breast cancer and familial breast cancer resulted in identification of an OR of developing breast cancer of about 2.6 which increased to about 4.6 if there were affected family members [59].

4.4   Breast Cancer Susceptibility Genes

The genetic basis of breast cancer is heterogeneous. Family studies, linkage analysis, case–control studies, genome-wide association studies (GWAS), and now whole-exome studies have revealed that there are germline mutations and variants of varying frequencies and significance involved in breast cancer. These gene changes are classified as high, moderate, and low penetrant with "penetrance" meaning the probability of developing breast cancer based on carrying a specific germline mutation. These include rare germline mutations associated with high penetrance (relative risks greater than 5), infrequent germline mutations associated with moderate penetrance (relative risks of about 1.5–5), and frequent common genetic variations each associated with low penetrance (relative risk less than 1.5). It is considered unlikely that additional high penetrant germline mutations remain to be identified. Genetic studies are now focusing on polygenic models in which risk varies based on combination of genotype and nongenetic factors such as environment and lifestyle choices.

4.5 High-Risk Genes

Six genes are associated with very high risks for developing breast cancer. The five genetic syndromes represented by these six genes are highly penetrant as overall lifetime breast cancer risk ranges from 45 to 85 % and are associated with variable expressivity and follow autosomal dominant inheritance. All female mutation carriers require increase surveillance for breast cancer beginning as young adults and for other cancers depending upon the underlying genetic condition.

4.5.1 BRCA1/BRCA2

BRCA1 was first reported in Fall 1994 and *BRCA2* 1 year later. Over the past 20 years, much research has been performed regarding the spectrum of associated cancers, lifetime risk for developing cancer, modifiers of risk, medical management options, and psychological issues. *BRCA1* and *BRCA2* germline mutations are now synonymous with the hereditary breast and ovarian cancer syndrome (HBOC). More than 3800 distinct pathogenic mutations have been reported [34]. Carrier frequency does vary between ethnic groups [21]. In the US non-Hispanic population, carrier frequency has been estimate to be about 1 in 400 [60].

Female carriers have a lifetime breast cancer risk of 50–85 % with a high risk for developing breast cancer prior to age 50. Risk for developing a second primary breast cancer is about 40–50 %. Epithelial ovarian cancer risk overall is about 10–40 % with BRCA1 mutations conferring a higher risk, 25–40 % [34].

Male BRCA2 carriers have about a 7–8 % lifetime risk of developing breast cancer and an increased risk for prostate cancer, especially aggressive tumors under the age of 65. Male BRCA1 mutation carriers may have an increased lifetime risk of about 1–2 % for developing breast cancer and an increased risk for developing prostate cancer [34].

Other associated cancers include fallopian tube and primary peritoneal carcinomas and pancreatic adenocarcinoma. Other cancers which may be associated include cutaneous and ocular melanoma and gastric, gallbladder, and bile duct cancers.

Predictors of *BRCA1* or *BRCA2* involvement include early average age of breast cancer diagnosis, presence of epithelial ovarian cancer, presence of male breast cancer, presence of a family member with both primary breast and primary epithelial ovarian cancer, triple-negative (ER-negative, PR-negative, HER2-negative) breast cancer, and being of Ashkenazi Jewish descent. Families described as having hereditary site-specific breast cancer, i.e., no epithelial ovarian cancer, are less likely to be identified with an underlying segregating *BRCA1* or *BRCA2* mutation. Mutation probability models have been developed. BRCAPRO (http://bcb.dfci. harvard.edu/bayesmendel/brcapro.php) and BOADICEA (Breast and Ovarian Analysis of Disease Incidence and Carrier Estimation Algorithm, http://ccge. medschl.cam.ac.uk/boadicea/) are both complex statistical analyses based on Bayesian analysis and incorporating all first- and second-degree relatives, ages, and whether affected or unaffected. Both of these models may be utilized for unaffected and affected patients. Tyrer–Cusick (http://www.ems-trials.org/riskevaluator/) is another model but is limited to unaffected individuals.

4.5.2   *TP53*

Inherited *TP53* mutations underlie Li–Fraumeni syndrome (LFS). The *TP53* gene, referred to as the "guardian of the genome," encodes a protein integral in cell cycle control. More than 750 distinct germline mutations have been identified in families with LFS [32]. Li–Fraumeni syndrome was suggested in 1969 by Drs. Li and Fraumeni after following the families of their pediatric patients with bone and soft-tissue sarcoma. The classic definition (Table 4.3) is an individual diagnosed with a sarcoma prior to age 45 who has a first-degree relative diagnosed with any cancer prior to age 45 and an additional first- or second-degree relative (in the same lineage) with any cancer diagnosed prior to 45 or with a sarcoma diagnosed at any age. Approximately 50–77 % of patients meeting the classic definition are identified with an underlying *TP53* germline mutation [4, 56]. Differing sets of genetic testing criteria have been suggested over the years leading to the use of "Li–Fraumeni-like syndrome." The Chompret criteria, first published in 2001 and revised in 2009 (Table 4.3), were associated with a 21 % detection rate in a 2010 study of 180 families suspected of having Li–Fraumeni syndrome [42].

The core component tumors associated with germline *TP53* mutations are early-onset breast cancer, soft-tissue sarcomas, osteosarcomas, adrenocortical carcinoma, and brain malignancies. Cancer-specific risk estimates have been difficult to determine, in part due to the rarity of the condition and range of tumors developing in these families. Ruijs et al. reported in their 2010 study a relative risk of 6.4 for female breast cancer [42]. Female *TP53* mutation carriers appear to have an overall higher lifetime risk for developing cancer, in comparison to male carriers, seemingly due to the breast cancer risk. Male breast cancer has rarely been reported. Ruijs et al. also reported that about one-third of the malignancies developing in the 24 families identified with a segregating *TP53* mutation were not core tumors. These other tumors included gastrointestinal and genitourinary cancers, melanoma, bronchoalveolar lung cancer, and non-medullary thyroid cancer [42].

TP53-associated malignancies often are diagnosed at young ages. About 50 % of cancers develop prior to age 30 years [4, 42]. Penetrance is very high with 90–100 %

Table 4.3 Li–Fraumeni syndrome (LFS)

Classic definition	Individual diagnosed with a sarcoma prior to age 45
	A first-degree relative (FDR) diagnosed with cancer prior to age 45
	An additional FDR or second-degree relative (SDR) (in the same lineage) with cancer diagnosed prior to 45 or with a sarcoma diagnosed at any age
Chompret criteria, revised	An individual diagnosed with a tumor belonging to the LFS tumor spectrum before age 46 (soft-tissue sarcoma, osteosarcoma, brain tumor, premenopausal breast cancer, adrenocortical carcinoma, leukemia, lung bronchoalveolar)
	At least one FDR or SDR with an LFS tumor (not breast cancer, if the proband has breast cancer) before age 56 or multiple primary tumors
	Or
	An individuals with multiple primary tumors (except multiple breast cancer), two of which belong to the LFS spectrum and the first of which was diagnosed before age 46
	Or
	An individual with adrenal cortical carcinoma or choroid plexus tumor, irrespective of family history

of *TP53* mutation carriers developing cancer by age 60 [43]. Affected individuals are at high risk for developing multiple primary tumors. The NCCN Clinical Practice Guidelines in Oncology, Genetic/Familial High-Risk Assessment: Breast and Ovarian Cancer (www.nccn.org) provide genetic testing criteria and management recommendations which are reviewed and revised annually [30].

4.5.3   PTEN

Diagnosis of *PTEN* hamartomatous tumor syndrome (PHTS) results upon identification of a germline *PTEN* mutation. *PTEN* mutations historically underlie approximately 85 % of patients clinically diagnosed with Cowden syndrome. However, a prospective study of 3399 patients meeting relaxed International Cowden Consortium criteria resulted in a *PTEN* germline mutation yield of only 8.8 % [53]. *PTEN* germline mutations also underlie Bannayan–Riley–Ruvalcaba syndrome, Proteus syndrome, and Proteus-like syndrome, each a complex congenital disorder.

Female *PTEN* mutation carriers have a significantly increased lifetime risk for developing breast cancer. Historically, this risk was 25–50 %. A recent prospective study found a 50 % risk by age 50 and an 85 % lifetime risk [53]. Female carriers are also at significant risk for benign breast tumors and benign and malignant tumors of the uterus. Male breast cancer has rarely been reported. *PTEN* mutation carriers are at increased risk for benign and malignant thyroid tumors, renal and colon cancer, and melanoma [53].

Table 4.4 Cowden syndrome (CS) diagnostic criteria

Pathognomonic criteria
Adult Lhermitte–Duclos disease (LDD), defined as the presence of a cerebellar dysplastic gangliocytoma
Mucocutaneous lesions, including facial trichilemmomas and facial/oral papillomas
Acral keratoses
Major criteria
Breast cancer
Epithelial thyroid cancer (non-medullary), especially follicular thyroid cancer
Macrocephaly (occipital frontal circumference ≥97th percentile – 58 cm for women, 60 cm for men)
Endometrial carcinoma
Minor criteria
Other thyroid lesions (e.g., adenoma, multinodular goiter)
Intellectual disability (IQ ≤75)
Hamartomatous intestinal polyps
Fibrocystic disease of the breast
Lipomas
Fibromas
Genitourinary tumors (especially renal cell carcinoma)
Genitourinary malformation
Uterine fibroids
An operational diagnosis of CS is made if an individual meets any one of the following criteria:
Pathognomonic mucocutaneous lesions combined with one of the following:
Six or more facial papules, of which three or more must be trichilemmoma
Cutaneous facial papules and oral mucosal papillomatosis
Oral mucosal papillomatosis and acral keratoses
Six or more palmoplantar keratoses
Two or more major criteria
One major and three or more minor criteria
Four or more minor criteria
In a family in which one individual meets the diagnostic criteria for CS listed above, other relatives are considered to have a diagnosis of CS if they meet any one of the following criteria:
The pathognomonic criteria
Any one major criterion with or without minor criteria
Two minor criteria
History of Bannayan–Riley–Ruvalcaba syndrome

Diagnostic criteria for Cowden syndrome have been established (Table 4.4). An online scoring system was developed based on more than 3300 prospective cases to assist in determining clinical utility of *PTEN* genetic testing, http://www.lerner.ccf.org/gmi/ccscore/ [52]. The NCCN Clinical Practice Guidelines in Oncology, Genetic/Familial High-Risk Assessment: Breast and Ovarian Cancer (www.nccn.org) provide genetic testing criteria and management recommendations which are reviewed and revised annually [30].

4.5.4 CDH1

Germline *CDH1* mutations result in hereditary diffuse gastric cancer and are associated with significantly increased risk for lobular breast cancer. Female *CDH1* mutation carriers have about an 83 % lifetime risk for developing diffuse gastric cancer (DGC) and about a 39–52 % lifetime risk for developing lobular breast cancer [22, 35]. Women presenting with early-onset lobular breast cancer and/or familial lobular breast cancer, with no known gastric cancer, have infrequently been identified with a germline *CDH1* mutation. In 2011, Schrader et al. reported on 318 cases of early-onset lobular or familial lobular breast cancer with no loss-of-function *CDH1* mutations and four non-synonymous variants (mutation alters the amino acid encoded) which possibly may be pathogenic [45]. There have since been a handful of cases published suggesting that *CDH1* genetic testing may be considered in the case of multiple lobular breast cancers. In a case report, Xie et al. reported two families with familial lobular breast cancer in which a *CDH1* mutation was identified [62]. Benusiglio et al. reported three unrelated women diagnosed with bilateral lobular breast cancer under the age of 50 who at the time had no family history of DGC but who later developed diffuse gastric cancer and were identified with *CDH1* germline mutations; the authors suggest *CDH1* testing should be considered in early-onset bilateral lobular breast cancer cases as the lobular breast cancer could be the presenting symptom in some families [3]. Interestingly, a recent study of bilateral lobular carcinoma in situ (LCIS) identified loss-of-function mutations in *CDH1* in 8 % (4 of 50 cases) of the study population though studies of unilateral LCIS have not [33].

4.5.5 STK11

STK11 germline mutations result in Peutz–Jeghers syndrome, a hamartomatous polyposis condition increasing the risk for a range of benign and malignant tumors, including breast cancer, and associated with a characteristic mucocutaneous pigmentation pattern. Female *STK11* mutation carriers have about an 8 and 32 % risk for developing breast cancer by ages 40 and 60, respectively [17].

4.6 Moderate-Risk Genes

In 2002, *BRCA2* was determined to be one of the genes underlying Fanconi anemia, a heterogeneous autosomal recessive condition [19]. This discovery led to analysis of other genes involved in Fanconi anemia resulting in identification of three other genes (*PALB2*, *BRIP1*, *RAD51C*) associated with moderately elevating breast cancer risk. Additional moderate-risk genes have been identified by similarly applying the candidate gene approach.

There remain a number of clinical limitations and questions:

1. There are significant deficiencies in the knowledge regarding the clinical implications of carrying a germline mutation in a moderate-risk gene, including the associated spectrum of cancers, the lifetime risk of developing cancer, and the age at which the risk of cancer begins to increase.
2. There are relatively few published case-controlled studies.
3. Evidence-based clinical management guidelines are not available, including what age to start screening, what screening tools are effective, and frequency.
4. Few family segregation studies have been completed and those that have been done document incomplete segregation in some cases, e.g., the breast cancers in the family and segregation of the identified mutation do not always coincide. As a result, the question, what is the lifetime cancer risk for the sister who did not inherit the mutation in her affected sister, is difficult to answer.
5. There may be significant differences in carrier frequency between ethnic groups and in cancer risks due to nongenetic modifiers present in different ethnic groups.
6. Do loss-of-function mutations and missense mutations confer similar or different cancer risks?

The following genes are currently included in many multigene panels:

4.6.1 PALB2

PALB2 encodes a protein which interacts with BRCA1 and BRCA2 and was first reported in 2006 as increasing breast cancer risk in British familial breast cancer cases [37]. Segregation analysis provided an initial relative risk of about 2.3 for developing breast cancer. Multiple subsequent studies have confirmed it to be associated with a moderate to possibly high risk for developing breast cancer with risk ranging from two- to sixfold. *PALB2* mutations appear to account for about 1–2 % of familial breast cancer. As noted earlier, lifetime cancer risk appears to be influenced by the extent of the family history.

4.6.2 ATM

The *ATM* gene underlies ataxia-telangiectasia (AT), an autosomal recessive disorder defined by neurologic deterioration, telangiectasias, immunodeficiency, increased rates of infection, and hypersensitivity to ionizing radiation. Approximately 0.5–1 % of the general population may be a heterozygous carrier of an *ATM* mutation [12, 40, 51]. Initial studies exploring breast cancer risk in *ATM* carriers provided conflicting results. But then in 2006, Renwick et al. reported on 443 UK familial breast cancer families and identified a relative risk of about 2.3 for breast cancer in carriers of AT-causing *ATM* mutations, which typically are truncating or splice-site mutations [40]. Subsequent studies have reported some missense mutations, primarily those acting through a dominant-negative effect, to confer an increased risk of varying levels. One example is the c.7271 T>G mutation which has repeatedly been found to confer as much as an eight-fold increased risk [14]. Further studies are needed to determine if breast cancer risk is defined by mutation type and/or location. Evidence-based clinical guidelines for managing risk for an asymptotic carrier are not available. Expert opinion is to manage risk based on personal risk factors and family history.

4.6.3 CHEK2

The CHEK2 protein is involved in the same pathway as the *BRCA1* and *TP53* proteins and is activated in response to DNA damage. One specific mutation, 1100delC, was established as a breast cancer risk factor in 2002 [26]. In Eastern and Northern European populations, the allele frequency in the general population is 0.2–1.4 % and nearly nonexistent in other populations including Chinese, Japanese, Brazilian, and Southern Europe. In the North American population, carrier frequency is about 0.3 % [31]. Several studies have shown that breast cancer risk is modified by the extent of family history. As already noted, Weischer and colleagues reported their meta-analysis of the *CHEK2* 1100delC mutation in early-onset breast cancer and familial breast cancer finding an OR of developing breast cancer of about 2.6 which increased to about 4.6 if there were affected family members [59]. Cybulski and colleagues reported similar results in their study of Polish familial breast cancer finding that risk increased from an OR of 3.3 if no family history to 5.0 if one affected first- or second-degree relative to 7.3 if there were both an affected first- and an affected second-degree relative. Additionally, they found that truncating mutations, of which 1100delC is one, confers a higher relative risk for breast cancer than the Polish missense founder mutation [9]. Multiple other *CHEK2* germline mutations have been identified, but for most, mutation-specific breast cancer risk estimates are not available. Clinical impact of identifying a germline *CHEK2* mutation in an unaffected woman appears to at least depend on mutation type, family history, and ancestry. Evidence-based clinical guidelines for managing risk for an asymptotic carrier are not available. Expert opinion is to manage risk based on personal risk factors and family history.

4.6.4 BRIP1

BRIP1 encodes a protein which interacts with BRCA1 and was first reported as increasing breast cancer risk twofold in British familial breast cancer cases in 2006 [46]. Nine (0.7 %) of 1212 familial breast cancer cases and 2 (0.09 %) of 2081 controls were identified with *BRIP1* truncating mutations. Genotyping of relatives was performed in four families; breast cancer phenotype did not completely segregate with *BRIP1* genotype. Overall, *BRIP1* germline mutations appear to be a rare cause of breast cancer. One of 70 Australian familial breast cancer cases was identified a *BRIP1* truncating mutation [61]. Separate studies of Finnish families with hereditary breast and ovarian cancer and of Russian breast cancer cases demonstrating features of hereditary cancer identified no *BRIP1* mutations [23, 49]. More recent data indicate the greater concern for female *BRIP1* mutations carriers may be for ovarian cancer [29, 36]. Evidence-based clinical guidelines for managing risk for an asymptotic carrier are not available. Expert opinion is to manage risk based on personal risk factors and family history.

4.6.5   *BARD1*

The possible involvement of *BARD1* germline mutations in familial breast cancer was first suggested in 1998 by Thai and colleagues [54]. Studies of familial *BRCA1/2*-negative breast cancer with and without ovarian cancer have identified *BARD1* mutations in a small percentage of cases. De Brakeleer and colleagues reported 3 (1.5 %) possible pathogenic mutations in 196 Belgian high-risk breast cancer families [1]. Ratajska and colleagues identified 3 (2.7 %) sequence variants suspected to be pathogenic in 109 high-risk Polish families [38]. On the other hand, no BARD1 mutations were identified in an Australian series of familial breast cancer. Clinical impact on cancer risk in asymptomatic carriers remains undefined.

4.6.6   *NF1*

Neurofibromatosis type 1 (NF1) is a common autosomal dominant condition predisposing to café au lait spots, neurofibromas, axillary and inguinal region freckling, malignant nerve sheath tumors, and central nervous system gliomas. Incidence is about 1 in 3500 worldwide. In 2005, Sharif et al. reported an increased incidence of breast cancer especially prior to age 50 in their cohort [48]. In 2012, Wang et al. reported similar findings in their Detroit, Michigan population [58]. Seminog and Goldacre calculated a relative risk of 6.5 for English female NF1 patients ages 30–39, of 4.4 for ages 40–49, and of 2.6 for ages 50–59 [47]. Interestingly, there have been at least two independent case reports of women developing early-onset breast cancer and carrying both a deleterious NF1 and deleterious *BRCA1* mutation.

4.6.7   *MRE11/RAD50/NBN*

These three proteins form the MRN protein complex and act in concert in response to DNA breakage. One specific *NBN* mutation, 657del5, is a founder mutation in the Slavic population and appears to confer a relative risk for breast cancer of about 2.5–3 [50]. A Finnish *RAD50* founder mutation, c. 687delT, was first reported to confer increased risk but subsequent data have been conflicting [18, 55]. *MRE11* mutations were first reported two of eight Danish breast cancer cases. Damiola and colleagues identified 9 (0.6 %) (1 *MRE11*, 4 *RAD50*, 4 *NBN*) truncating or splice-junction mutations out of 1312 early-onset breast cancers as well as 20 (1.5 %) rare missense mutations which were considered possibly pathogenic [10]. Clinical impact on breast cancer risk in asymptomatic carriers remains undefined.

4.6.8   *RAD51C*

The first association between cancer risk and *RAD51C* germline mutations was published in 2010 [27]. Meindl et al. reported on 1100 German families, 620 with breast cancer and 480 with breast and ovarian cancer. No germline *RAD51C* mutations were identified in the breast cancer only families, and 6 (1.3 %) *RAD51C* mutations were identified in the 480 breast/ovarian cancer families. Germline *RAD51C* mutations appear to be a rare cause of familial breast cancer. Of 70 Australian familial breast cancer cases, none were identified as a *RAD51C* mutation [62]. Of 95 Russian breast cancer cases demonstrating features of hereditary cancer and of 108 breast cancer cases diagnosed before age 35, none were identified with a *RAD51C* mutation. Its strongest association appears to be with ovarian cancer [8, 25]. Currently, there are no evidence-based clinical management guidelines available for *RAD51C* mutation carriers.

4.6.9   *RAD51D*

As with *RAD51C* germline mutations, *RAD51D* mutations principally appear to increase risk for ovarian carcinoma. The first report of *RAD51D* germline mutations and cancer risk was published in 2011 [24]. Loveday et al. reported on 911 probands, all of whom were affected members of families with breast and ovarian and having tested negative for *BRCA1* and BRCA2. Eight (0.9 %) germline mutations were identified as having a strong association with ovarian cancer. Four mutations were found in the 235 families with two or more ovarian cancers, and three (5 %) mutations were identified in the 59 families with three or more ovarian cancers. A strong association with breast cancer was not identified. They studied an additional 737 unrelated probands from families with familial breast cancer with no *RAD51D* mutations being identified. Of 171 Spanish familial breast cancer probands, none were identified with a *RAD51D* mutation though 4 of 491 (0.8 %) probands from families with breast and ovarian cancer were identified with a *RAD51D* mutation [15]. Currently, there are no evidence-based clinical management guidelines available for *RAD51D* mutation carriers.

4.7 Associated Autosomal Recessive Conditions

Several of these genes when mutations are present in the homozygous (both alleles contain the same germline mutation) or compound heterozygous state (both alleles contain a germline mutation, also referred to as biallelic mutations) cause autosomal recessive conditions (Tables 4.5 and 4.6). A family history of one of these conditions may impact decisions on genetic testing. Alternatively, identification of a germline mutation indicates possible reproductive implications which need to be addressed (see Sect. 4.13.1).

BRCA2, *PALB2*, *BRIP1*, and *RAD51C* each result in a subtype of Fanconi anemia. Fanconi anemia is a heterogeneous disorder with 15 genes identified and characterized by progressive bone marrow failure, increased risk for leukemia and solid tumors, myelodysplastic syndrome, and increased risk for physical abnormalities including short stature, abnormalities of thumb and forearms, microcephaly, and hypogonadism [1]. Incidence is about 1 in 360,000 live births. Estimated carrier frequency is about 1 in 300 although some populations, including the Ashkenazi Jewish, Spanish Gypsy, and sub-Saharan African, have carrier frequencies closer to 1 in 100.

ATM mutations underlie ataxia-telangiectasia which is typically characterized by progressive cerebellar ataxia beginning between ages 1 and 4 years resulting in most individuals becoming wheelchair-bound by adolescence. Affected individuals also demonstrate slurred speech, chorea, telangiectasias of the conjunctivae, immunodeficiency, frequent infections, and an increased risk for malignancy, particularly leukemia and lymphoma. Affected individuals are unusually sensitive to ionizing radiation. Incidence in the United States is about 1 in 40,000–100,000 live births [13].

Table 4.5 Breast cancer susceptibility: possible levels of information

	High-risk genes	Moderate-risk genes	Newly described genes
Genes	BRCA1, BRCA2, CDH1, PTEN, STK11, TP53	ATM, CHEK2, NF1, PALB2	BARD1, BRIP1, MRE11A, NBN, RAD50, RAD51C, RAD51D
Lifetime breast cancer risk	45–85 %	Relative risk of 2–5; cancer risk becoming more defined	Not well defined Relative risk of 1.5–3
Medical management	Established guidelines for screening and prevention	Evidence-based guidelines not established; management based on age and family history	Evidence-based guidelines not established; difficult to make recommendations due to poor understanding of gene; management based on age and family history
Implications to family	Straightforward, well defined	Less well defined	Not well defined

Table 4.6 Associated autosomal recessive conditions

Gene	Autosomal recessive condition	Features
BRCA2	Fanconi anemia, type D1	Progressive bone marrow failure, increased risk for leukemia, myelodysplastic syndrome, and solid tumors, short stature, pigmentation abnormalities, abnormalities of thumb and forearms, microcephaly, microphthalmia, structural renal anomalies, and hypogonadism
BRIP1	Fanconi anemia, type J	
PALB2	Fanconi anemia, type N	
RAD51C	Fanconi anemia, type O	
ATM	Ataxia-telangiectasia	Progressive cerebellar ataxia, involuntary movements, immunodeficiency, increased frequency of infections, increased risk for malignancy, and especially leukemia and lymphoma, sensitive to ionizing radiation
NBN	Nijmegen breakage syndrome	Microcephaly, growth retardation, short stature, recurrent respiratory infections, increased risk for lymphoma, mild–moderate intellectual disability, premature ovarian failure

NBN mutations result in Nijmegen breakage syndrome which is characterized by progressive microcephaly, growth retardation, short stature, recurrent respiratory infections, increased risk for lymphoma, and normal development for the first of life followed by regression with many demonstrating mild–moderate intellectual disability by adolescence. Estimated incidence of Nijmegen breakage syndrome is unknown but estimated to be approximately 1 in a 100,000, though it is more common in the Eastern European/Slavic population group where the carrier frequency of a common mutation may be as high as 1 in 155 [57].

4.8 Genetic Testing

Clinical genetic testing for breast cancer susceptibility principally became available in 1996 after the identification of the *BRCA1* gene in 1994 and of the *BRCA2* gene in 1995. Several modifications to methodology occurred, 5-site rearrangement panel in the late 1990s and BART in 2006. More significant changes started in March 2012 when Ambry Genetics became the first commercial laboratory to market a multigene panel for breast cancer susceptibility. Multigene panels came about due to the development of next-generation (next-gen) sequencing technology, also known as massively parallel sequencing. A primary benefit of these newer laboratory techniques was the cost savings of testing many genes for about the same cost as testing two or three genes. Timeliness, or turnaround time, has in some cases offered a significant improvement in patient care, especially in cases where the differential includes several genes. Previously, genes would have to be tested in sequence. Perhaps one of the most significant event occurred in June 2013, the Supreme Court invalidated portions of Myriad Genetic Laboratories' patent claims involving

BRCA1 and *BRCA2*, which permitted other laboratories to offer *BRCA1* and *BRCA2* genetic testing.

Genetic testing options now include single gene/genetic condition such as *TP53* or HBOC (*BRCA1/BRCA2* analysis) and multigene panels of which there are many versions including "high-risk gene panels" consisting of five or six of the well-described high-risk breast cancer conditions as well as more extensive panels of 17, 21, or 25 genes.

Reasons for considering genetic testing are multiple and may be impacted by the age of the patient, strength of her family history, and her motivation/purpose in assessing her lifetime cancer risk. In the case of assessing a patient presenting due to a family history of breast cancer, it is important to assess whether an affected family member is available and, if so, interested in undergoing genetic evaluation and testing, in order to more fully evaluate the possible involvement of an underlying genetic predisposition. Involving the family member most likely to carry a germline mutation provides the most information about whether an underlying genetic cause is present and is the most cost-effective approach.

Case Example
A 30-year-old healthy patient has a family history of breast cancer which could be secondary to a *BRCA1* or *BRCA2* mutation. If the patient undergoes *BRCA1/2* testing and no mutation identified, her lifetime breast cancer risk remains at least moderately elevated. On the other hand, if her affected mother undergoes *BRCA1/2* genetic testing and no mutation identified, it has been documented that the mother's breast cancer is not due to a known genetic mutation and there is no medical need for the patient (and any sisters she may have) to undergo genetic testing. Her medical management though will continue to be based on her family history. If, however, her mother tests positive for a germline *BRCA2* mutation, the patient can undergo focused *BRCA2* genetic testing, at a fraction of the cost of comprehensive *BRCA1/2* analysis, and definitively learn whether or not she inherited the familial risk for breast cancer. If testing negative for the mutation identified in her mother, her lifetime breast cancer risk would return to general population level, barring any other personal risk factors.

If there is sufficient concern for an underlying genetic predisposition and if an affected family member is not available or is not interested, unaffected patients may choose to undergo genetic testing. It is important to counsel that the absence of a germline mutation will not reduce the lifetime cancer risk to the general population and there may be a higher frequency of ambiguous (genetic variant of uncertain significance) results.

Table 4.7 outlines the five possible results when performing genetic testing when no familial mutation has been identified.

Table 4.7 Gene analysis: possible results

Result	Interpretation	Impact on management
Pathogenic (deleterious)	Associated with increased risk for developing cancer	Medical management is based on the associated syndrome's guidelines
Genetic variant, likely pathogenic	Current clinical and molecular evidence indicates a high, but not conclusive, likelihood that the variant is deleterious	
Genetic variant, uncertain clinical significance	Current clinical and molecular evidence is inconclusive	No impact on medical management; management is based on personal/family history; depending on extent of family history, underlying genetic predisposition may still be present
Genetic variant, likely benign	Current clinical and molecular evidence indicates a high, but not conclusive, likelihood that the variant is benign	Management is based on personal/family history; depending on extent of family history, underlying genetic predisposition may still be present
Benign (no mutation identified)	No association with an increased risk for developing cancer	

4.9 Genetic Testing When a Familial Mutation Has Been Identified

For patients who report a family history of a germline mutation, focused (single-site) genetic testing is available. To order focused genetic testing, a copy of the family member's genetic test report is required, firstly, to confirm a deleterious mutation was identified and, secondly, to inform the laboratory which mutation is to be tested for; thirdly, genetic testing best practices include using the same laboratory for familial testing to minimize the possibility of a false-negative result.

Focused genetic testing often is relatively straightforward; however, there are several potential pitfalls. A detailed three-generation pedigree and documentation of ancestry remain important as is documenting the degree of relationship between the patient and the family member identified with the germline mutation. Although testing negative for a high-risk germline mutation present in a biological relative indicates the patient does not carry that familial risk factor for developing breast cancer, if the family member is a distant relative and intervening affected family members have not tested (Fig. 4.2), it may be difficult to conclude that the patient's lifetime breast cancer risk has been reduced to general population level. If the family member is the patient's mother, but there are several paternal relatives treated for breast cancer, the patient's risk may still be elevated (Fig. 4.3). If the patient has Ashkenazi Jewish ancestry in the opposite lineage from the one in which the mutation is segregating, she may still have an increased risk if she was not also tested for the BRCA1/2 Ashkenazi Jewish founder mutations. The patient's lifetime

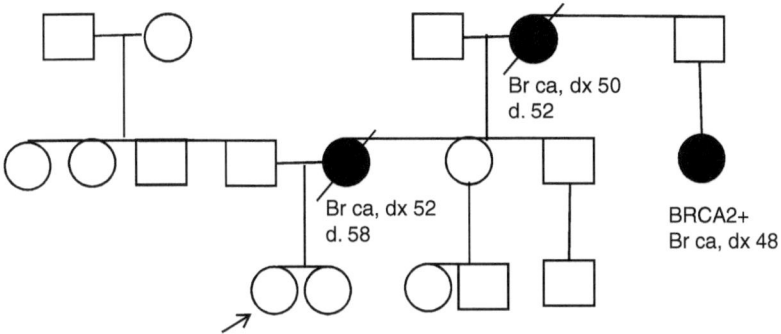

Fig. 4.2 A 30-year-old patient, tested negative for BRCA2 mutation in mother's maternal cousin. Without genetic data for her biologically closer maternal relatives, it is difficult to state that her lifetime risk has been reduced to general population level. Further actions which could assist in determination of her breast cancer risk include (1) her sister and maternal aunt/uncle or cousins testing, and if positive for the identified mutation, this information would clarify the mother's BRCA2 status and/or (2) obtaining more information from mother's maternal extended family to clarify if the mother's affected cousin inherited the mutation from her father (the mother's biological uncle) or her mother (the mother's nonbiological aunt). Key: *circle* female, *square* male, *colored-in* diagnosed with breast cancer, *arrow* indicates the patient

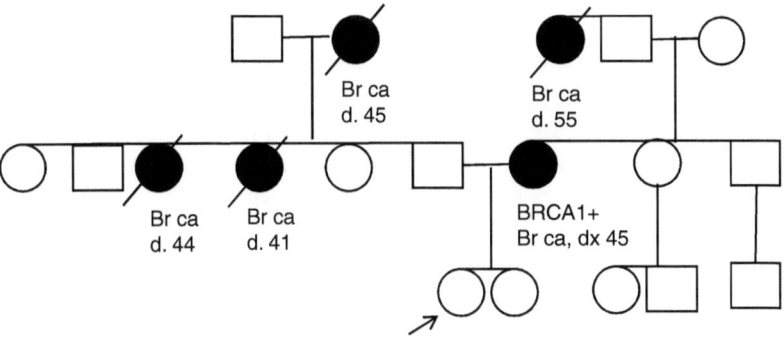

Fig. 4.3 A 30-year-old patient, tested negative for BRCA1 mutation identified in mother. Her lifetime risk cannot be reduced to general population level due to paternal family history of breast cancer. Key: *circle* female, *square* male, *colored-in* diagnosed with cancer, *arrow* indicates the patient

breast cancer risk may still be elevated if other personal risk factors, i.e., atypical ductal hyperplasia, are present.

With the advent of multigene panel testing, unaffected patients are presenting with family histories of moderately penetrant genes and/or of newly described genes. In these cases, focused genetic testing may or may not impact the patient's medical care, especially in the case of newly described genes. Testing negative for the identified germline mutation may not indicate that the patient's lifetime risk for developing breast cancer is reduced to general population level as these types of studies have not been completed. Additionally, as breast cancer risk appears to be modified, in some cases by strength of family history, involvement of other risk factors is probable but currently unknown.

> **Case Example**
> A 54-year-old unaffected woman reports her 56-year-old sister was treated for breast cancer at 48 and tested positive for a *BARD1* mutation. Their maternal aunt developed breast cancer at age 60; she has not undergone genetic testing for breast cancer susceptibility. There is no other family history of cancer. *BARD1* germline mutations may increase risk for developing breast cancer about twofold. She tests negative for the identified *BARD1* mutation; however, she cannot be informed to what degree her lifetime breast cancer risk has been reduced. She should continue to be followed based on her personal and family history.

4.10 Single Gene/Genetic Condition (*BRCA1/2*, *TP53*, *PTEN*) Genetic Testing Versus Multigene Panel Testing

Each case for which genetic testing for cancer susceptibility is medically relevant should be assessed independently for the extent of testing. Each case does not require a multigene panel, and even in cases for which a multigene panel may be reasonable, patients should be involved in the decision-making whether to proceed with single gene/genetic condition testing or multigene panel.

Multigene panels are associated with an increased frequency of variants of unknown clinical significance (VUS). Ambry Genetics, via their website, cite that nearly 22 % of their BreastNext (17 genes) results are VUS. Variants of unknown clinical significance are not necessarily benign and can be associated with harm. Increase anxiety and confusion may result on the part of patients and their family members. Misinterpretation by healthcare providers resulting in inappropriate medical recommendations has occurred.

With the advent of multigene panels, the possibility of incidental findings has arrived. A germline mutation may be identified in a gene not previously suspected. For example, a *TP53* mutation may be identified though the family history is not consistent with Li–Fraumeni syndrome or a *CDH1* mutation may be identified though the family is negative for diffuse gastric cancer. These are difficult situations. Li–Fraumeni syndrome is associated with cancer developing in childhood and young adulthood and affects multiple organs, which psychologically is very different from a diagnosis of HBOC. Standard management for *CDH1* germline mutations is prophylactic gastrectomy as screening for diffuse gastric cancer in known *CDH1* families has been shown to be ineffective.

There currently are no consensus guidelines indicting when to order multigene panels. The 2015 NCCN Clinical Practice Guidelines in Oncology, Genetic/Familial

High-Risk Assessment: Breast and Ovarian Cancer (www.nccn.org) addressed the use of these panels and noted the following [30]:

1. Patients who have a personal or family history consistent with a single gene/ genetic condition are best served by genetic testing for that specific genetic condition.
2. If more than one gene can explain an inherited genetic condition, a multigene panel may be more efficient and/or cost-effective.
3. There may be a role for using a multigene panel if the personal and/or family history strongly implicate a genetic etiology but prior testing for a single genetic condition was uninformative.

4.11 Informed Consent

Informed consent for genetic testing for breast cancer susceptibility is multifaceted and should include the following:

- Purpose of the test
- Voluntary nature of genetic testing
- Clinical utility
- Possible results including possibility of:

  False-negative result
  Inconclusive result (variant of unknown clinical significance)
  Incidental result

- Available medical management options including:

  Effectiveness/noneffectiveness (i.e., screening for epithelial ovarian cancer)
  Availability of consensus or evidence-based guidelines

- Possible emotional consequences, e.g., anger, distress, guilt, decreased self-esteem, due to:

  Documentation of increased cancer risk and consequent need to increase screening and/or consideration of risk-reducing surgeries
  The inability to predict one's future health based solely on gene status
  "Being spared" the familial risk
  Possible changes in family relationships
  Development of tension due to differing perspectives on genetic testing and/or medical management choices
  Discovery of previously unknown biological relationships (adoption, nonpaternity)

- Possible psychosocial consequences, status of genetic nondiscrimination laws, and employment protections
- Implications on one's immediate and extended family:

  Inheritance risk to children, siblings, a parent, and extended family

4.12 Considerations When Choosing a Laboratory

There are now multiple laboratories in the United States offering *BRCA1* and
BRCA2 gene analysis as well as multigene panels. These include commercial and
academic laboratories. Cost, turnaround time, and level of service can be significantly
different. Considerations should include:

- Documentation that the laboratory is CLIA-approved.
- What genes are available, either to be ordered singly or in multigene panels?
  What is the lab director's rationale for inclusion of genes?
- Documentation of methodology, including depth of coverage. Is Sanger
  sequencing used for confirmation of variants identified by next-gen sequencing?
  For reference, laboratory guidelines are available from the American College of
  Medical Genetics and Genomics [39].
- Process of classifying gene changes, i.e., what is the laboratory's basis for clas-
  sifying a gene change as deleterious? As a variant of unknown clinical signifi-
  cance? As a neutral polymorphism? Laboratory guidelines are available through
  the American College of Medical Genetic and Genomic [41].
- Is supporting evidence for the interpretation of the identified gene change readily
  available in the test report?
- What is the rate of variants of unknown clinical significance?
- Does the lab have a variant reclassification program? What does it consist of?
- Quality of customer support. Are medical directors and genetic counselors
  readily available? Some laboratories offer extra support such as pre-verification
  of insurance coverage, which technically is not important but lessens the burden
  on physicians and their staff.

When testing for a known familial mutation, it is best to utilize the same
laboratory. If a different laboratory is used, the laboratory may require a positive
control, to ensure their assay allows for identification of the familial mutation.
Different laboratories may use different probes. It is considered unlikely, but
possible, for a patient to carry a polymorphism which interferes with the annealing
of the probe resulting in a false-negative result.

4.13 Psychosocial/Familial Aspects

Genetic discrimination, defined as the misuse of genetic information, remains a
concern for some patients although this concern has decreased significantly from
the mid-1990s. The Genetic Information Nondiscrimination Act of 2008 (GINA)
signed by President George W. Bush is a federal law that protects against misuse of
genetic information by most medical insurers and employers.

GINA protects against medical insurers using or requiring genetic information in
decisions regarding eligibility for medical insurance and in establishing premiums
and terms of coverage. GINA protects against employers using genetic information

in making decisions regarding hiring, firing, promotion, and pay and in segregating or otherwise mistreating an employee. For example, an employer cannot collect family medical history in pre-employment medical examinations. Family medical information, though, may become known to an employer through voluntary employer-sponsored wellness programs or through Family and Medical Leave Act (FMLA) forms but GINA prohibits the employer from misusing this information. GINA's employment protections do not cover small employers, those with fewer than 15 employees.

GINA provides protection for asymptomatic carriers of a germline mutation. GINA does not apply if the individual has developed manifestations of the genetic condition. Other federal laws such as the Affordable Care Act of 2010 (ACA), Health Insurance Portability and Accountability Act of 1996 (HIPPA), and the Americans with Disability Act (ADA) may apply once an individual has clinical symptoms of the genetic condition.

GINA does not apply to life insurance or disability or long-term insurance. It also does not apply to those in the US Military who are covered by Tricare, veterans who receive their medical care through the Veterans Administration, the Indian Health Service, and federal employees enrolled in the Federal Employee Health Benefits Plan. Federal employees receive protection from Executive Order 13,145 signed by President Bill Clinton in 2000 which disallows federal employers from requesting or requiring genetic information from their employees and in using genetic information in hiring and promotion decisions.

4.13.1 Familial Aspects

Identification of a germline mutation in an autosomal dominant condition documents that all first-degree relatives (parents, siblings, and children) each have a 50 % (1-in-2) chance for carrying the identified mutation. Second-degree relatives (half-siblings, nieces/nephews, aunts/uncles, grandparents) each have a 25 % (1-in-4) chance for carrying the identified mutation.

Determining whether the patient inherited the identified mutation from the mother or the father is not always clear. It is expected that, in the case of *BRCA1* and *BRCA2* mutations, a parent carries the identified mutation as de novo occurrences of *BRCA1* or *BRCA2* mutations have rarely been reported in the medical literature. In some cases, it is not possible to state whether the *BRCA1* or *BRCA2* mutation was inherited from the mother or father due to family structure, such as small family size or absence of multiple older women. Even if there is a history of breast cancer in one lineage, unless it is early-onset disease and there are multiple affected women, it may be red herring. If possible, it is best to test a parent in order to clarify in which lineage the mutation is segregating or, alternatively, an affected extended relative with the expected phenotype. If neither of these is possible, once an extended family member tests positive for the identified mutation, the at-risk lineage will be determined.

Predictive genetic testing for minor children is not recommended for adult-onset conditions, such as HBOC and *CDH1*, as changes to their medical care will not be implemented until at least young adulthood. Postponing focused genetic testing until young adulthood allows children to participate in the decision-making about learning their gene status. Adults who are at risk for carrying a germline mutation predisposing to cancer do not always choose to undergo genetic testing or choose to postpone it until after they have had their own children; therefore, parents who choose to test minor children for adult-onset conditions risk damaging their relationship with their children and the child's self-determination.

A side effect of utilizing multigene panels has been documentation of having children and grandchildren at risk for autosomal recessive conditions such as ataxia-telangiectasia and Fanconi anemia. Once a patient has been informed he/she is a carrier of a germline mutation in *ATM, NBN, BRCA2, BRIP1*, or *RAD51C*, counseling needs to include discussion of reproductive implications. If the patient is of childbearing age, there would be a 25 % chance for having a child affected by one of these conditions, if his/her reproductive partner was also a carrier of a germline mutation in the same gene. If the patient has children, counseling needs to include that each child could be a carrier (50 % chance) leading to the possibility of having grandchildren affected, if that child's reproductive partner also carried a germline mutation in the same gene. Carrier frequency of these mutations is based on the gene involved and ethnicity. Counseling may include the availability of preconceptional genetic counseling and alternative reproductive options.

References

1. Alter BP, Kupfer G. Fanconi anemia. 14 Feb 2002 [Updated 7 Feb 2013]. In: Pagon RA, Adam MP, Ardinger HH, et al., editors. GeneReviews® [Internet]. Seattle: University of Washington; 1993–2015. Available from: http://www.ncbi.nlm.nih.gov/books/NBK1401/.
2. Antoniou AC, Casadei S, Heikkinen T, Barrowdale D, Pylkäs K, Roberts J, et al. Breast cancer risk in families with mutations in PALB2. N Engl J Med. 2014;371:497–506.
3. Benusiglio PR, Malka D, Rouleau E, De Pauw A, Buecher B, Noguès C, et al. CDH1 germline mutations and the hereditary diffuse gastric and lobular breast cancer syndrome: a multicentre study. J Med Gen. 2013;50:486–9.
4. Birch JM, Hartley AL, Tricker KJ, Presser J, Condie A, Kelsey AM, et al. Prevalence and diversity of constitutional mutations in the p53 gene among 21 Li-Fraumeni families. Cancer Res. 1994;54:1298–304.
5. Bougeard G, Renaux-Petel M, Flaman JM, Charbonnier C, Fermey P, Belotti M, et al. Revisiting Li-Fraumeni syndrome from *TP53* mutation carriers. J Clin Oncolo. 2015;33:2345–52.
6. Calvez-Kelm FL, Javier O, Damiola F, Forey N, Robinot N, Durand G, et al. RAD51 and breast cancer susceptibility: No evidence for rare variant association in the Breast Cancer Family Registry Study. PLoS One. 2012;7:e52372. doi:10.1371/journal.pone.0052374
7. Cragun D, Camperlengo L, Robinson E, Caldwell M, Kim J, Phelan C, et al. Differences in *BRCA* counseling and testing practices based on ordering provider type. Genet Med. 2015; 17:51–7.
8. Coulet F, Frajac A, Colas C, Eyries M, Dion-Miniere A, Rouzier R, et al. Germline RAD51C mutations in ovarian cancer susceptibility. Clin Genet. 2013;83:332–6.

9. Cybulski C, Wokołorczyk D, Jakubowska A, Huzarski T, Byrski T, Gronwald J, et al. Risk of breast cancer in women with a CHEK2 mutation with and without a family history of breast cancer. J Clini Oncolo. 2011;29:3747–52.

10. Damiola F, Pertesi M, Oliver J, Le Calvez-Kelm F, Voegele C, Young EL, et al. Rare key functional domain missense substitutions in MRE11A, RAD50, and NBN contribute to breast cancer susceptibility: results from a Breast Cancer Family Registry case–control mutation-screening study. Breast Cancer Res. 2014;16:R58.

11. De Brakeleer S, De Grève J, Loris R, Janin N, Lissens W, Sermijn E, et al. Cancer Predisposing missense and protein truncating BARD1 mutations in non-BRCA1 or BRCA2 breast cancer families. Hum Mutat. 2010;31:E1175–85. doi:10.1002/humu.21200

12. FitzGerald MG, Bean JM, Hegde SR, Unsal H, MacDonald DJ, Harkin DP, et al. Heterozygous ATM mutations do not contribute to early onset of breast cancer. Nat Genet. 1997;15: 307–10.

13. Gatti R. Ataxia-telangiectasia. 19 Mar 1999 [Updated 11 May 2010]. In: Pagon RA, Adam MP, Ardinger HH, et al., editors. GeneReviews® [Internet]. Seattle: University of Washington; 1993–2015. Available from: http://www.ncbi.nlm.nih.gov/books/NBK26468/.

14. Goldgar DE, Healey S, Dowty JG, Da Silva L, Chen X, Spurdle AB, et al. Rare variants in the ATM gene and risk of breast cancer. Breast Cancer Res. 2011;13:R73.

15. Gutiérrez-Enríquez S, Bonache S, de Garibay GR, Osorio A, Santamariña M, Ramón y Cajal T. About 1% of the breast and ovarian Spanish families testing negative for BRCA1 and BRCA2 are carriers of RAD51D pathogenic variants. Int J of Can. 2013;134:2088–97.

16. Hampel H, Bennett RL, Buchanan A, Pearlman R, Wiesner GL, Guideline Development Group of the American College of Medical Genetics and Genomics Professional Practice and Guidelines Committee and of the National Society of Genetic Counselors Practice Guidelines Committee. A practice guideline from the American College of Medical Genetics and Genomics and the National Society of Genetic Counselors: referral indications for cancer predisposition assessment. Genet Med. 2014;17:70–87.

17. Hearle N, Schumacher V, Menko FH, Olschwang S, Boardman LA, Gille JJP, et al. Frequency and spectrum of cancers in the Peutz-Jeghers Syndrome. Clin Cancer Res. 2006;12:3209–15.

18. Heikkinen K, Rapakko K, Karppinen SM, Erkko H, Knuutila S, Lundan T, et al. RAD50 and NBS1 are breast cancer susceptibility genes associated with genomic instability. Carcinogenesis. 2006;27:1593–9.

19. Howlett NG, Taniguchi T, Olson S, Cox B, Waisfisz Q, De Die-Smulders C, et al. Biallelic inactivation of BRCA2 in Fanconi anemia. Science. 2002;297:606–9.

20. Iniesta MD, Gorin MA, Chien LC, Thomas SM, Milliron KJ, Douglas JA, et al. Absence of CHEK2*1100delC mutation in families with hereditary breast cancer in North America. Cancer Genet Cytogenet. 2010;15:136–40.

21. John EM, Miron A, Gong G, Phipps AI, Felberg A, Li FP, et al. Prevalence of pathogenic BRCA1 mutation carriers in 5 US racial/ethnic groups. JAMA. 2007;298:2869–76.

22. Kaurah P, MacMillan A, Boyd N, Senz J, De Luca A, Chun N, et al. Founder and recurrent CDH1 mutations in families with hereditary diffuse gastric cancer. JAMA. 2007;297:2360–72.

23. Kuusisto KM, Bebel A, Vihinen M, Schleutker J, Sallinen SL. Screening for BRCA1, BRCA2, CHEK2, PALB2, BRIP1, RAD50, and CDH1 mutations in high-risk Finnish BRCA1/2-founder mutation-negative breast and/or ovarian cancer individuals. Breast Cancer Res. 2011;13:R20.

24. Loveday C, Turnbull C, Ramsay E, Hughes D, Ruark E, Frankum JR, et al. Germline mutations in RAD51D confer susceptibility to ovarian cancer. Nat Genet. 2011;43:879–82.

25. Loveday C, Turnbull C, Ruark E, Xicola RMM, Ramsay E, Hughes D, et al. Germline RAD51C mutations confer susceptibility to ovarian cancer. Nat Genet. 2012;44:474–6.

26. Meijers-Heijboer H, van den Ouweland A, Klijn J, Wasielewski M, de Snoo A, Oldenburg R, et al. Nat Genet. Low penetrance susceptibility to breast cancer due to CHEK2 1100delC in noncarriers of BRCA1 or BRCA2 mutations. 2002;31:55–9

27. Meindl A, Hellebrand H, Wiek C, Erven V, Wappenschmidt B, Niederacher D, et al. Germline mutations in breast and ovarian cancer pedigrees establish RAD51C as a human cancer susceptibility gene. Nat Genet. 2010;42:410–4.
28. Miller CE, Krautscheid P, Baldwin EE, Tvrdik T, Openshaw AS, Hart K, et al. Genetic counselor review of genetic test orders in a reference laboratory reduces unnecessary testing. Am J Med Genet Part A. 2014;164A:1094–101.
29. Minion LE, Dolinsky JS, Chase DM, Dunlop CL, Chao EC, Monk BJ. Hereditary predisposition to ovarian cancer, looking beyond BRCA1/BRCA. Gynecol Oncol. 2015;137:86–92.
30. National Comprehensive Cancer Network [Internet]. NCCN clinical practice guidelines in oncology: genetic/familial high-risk assessment: breast and ovarian cancer. Ver 1.2015. Available from: http://www.nccn.org.
31. Offit K, Pierce H, Kirchhoff T, Kolachana P, Rapaport B, Gregersen P, et al. Frequency of CHEK2*1100delC in New York breast cancer cases and controls. BMC Med Genet. 2003;4:1.
32. Petitjean A, Mathe E, Kato S, Ishioka C, Tavtigian SV, Hainaut P, et al. Impact of mutant p53 functional properties on TP53 mutation patterns and tumor phenotype: lessons from recent developments in the IARC TP53 database. Hum Mutat. 2007;28:622–9. (database version: R17, November 2013).
33. Petridis SI, Kohut K, Gorman P, Caneppele M, Shah V, et al. Germline CDH1 mutations in bilateral lobular carcinoma in situ. Br J Can. 2014;110:1053–7.
34. Petrucelli N, Daly MB, Feldman GL. BRCA1 and BRCA2 hereditary breast and ovarian cancer. 4 Sep 1998 [Updated 26 Sep 2013]. In: Pagon RA, Adam MP, Ardinger HH, et al., editors. GeneReviews® [Internet]. Seattle: University of Washington; 1993–2015. Available from: http://www.ncbi.nlm.nih.gov/books/NBK1247/.
35. Pharoah PD, Guilford P, Caldas C. Incidence of gastric cancer and breast cancer in CDH1 (E-cadherin) mutation carriers from hereditary diffuse gastric cancer families. Gastroenterology. 2001;121:1348–53.
36. Rafnar T, Gudbjartsson DF, Sulem P, Jonasdottir A, Sigurdsson A, Jonasdottir A, et al. Mutations in BRIP1 confer high risk of ovarian cancer. Nat Genet. 2011;43:1104–7.
37. Rahman N, Seal S, Thompson D, Kelly P, Renwick A, Elliott A, Reid S, et al. PALB2, which encodes a BRCA2-interacting protein, is a breast cancer susceptibility gene. Nat Genet. 2006;39:165–7.
38. Ratajska M, Antoszewska E, Piskorz A, Brozek I, Borg Å, Kusmierek H, et al. Cancer predisposing BARD1 mutations in breast-ovarian cancer families. Breast Cancer Res Treat. 2012;131:89–97.
39. Rehm HL, Bale SJ, Bayrak-Toydemir P, Berg JS, Brown KK, Deignan JL, American College of Medical Genetic and Genomics Practice Guidelines, et al. ACMG clinical laboratory standards for next-generation sequencing. Genet Med. 2013;15:733–47.
40. Renwick A, Thompson D, Seal S, Kelly P, Chagtai T, Ahmed M, North B, et al. ATM mutations that cause ataxia-telangiectasia are breast cancer susceptibility alleles. Nat Genet. 2006;38:873–5.
41. Richards S, Aziz N, Bale S, Bick D, Das S, Gastier-Foster J, et al. Standards and guidelines for the interpretation of sequence variants: a joint consensus recommendations of the American College of Medical Genetics and Genomics and the Association for Molecular Pathology. Genet Med. 2015;17:405–22.
42. Ruijs MW, Verhoef S, Rookus MA, Pruntel R, van der Hout AH, Hogervorst FB, et al. TP53 germline mutation testing in 180 families suspected of Li-Fraumeni syndrome: mutation detection rate and relative frequency of cancers in different familial phenotypes. J of Med Genet. 2010;47:421–8.
43. Schneider KA, DiGianni LM, Patenaude AF, Klar N, Stopfer JE, Calzone KA, et al. Accuracy of cancer family histories: comparison of two breast cancer syndromes. Genet Test. 2004;8:222–8.

44. Schneider KA, Zelley K, Nichols KE, et al. Li-fraumeni syndrome. 19 Jan 1999 [Updated 11 Apr 2013]. In: Pagon RA, Adam MP, Ardinger HH, et al., editors. GeneReviews® [Internet]. Seattle: University of Washington; 1993–2015. Available from: http://www.ncbi.nlm.nih.gov/books/NBK1311/. Accessed 15 Jun 2015.

45. Schrader KA, Masciari S, Boyd N, Salamanca C, Senz J, Saunders DN, et al. Germline mutations in CDH1 are infrequent in women with early-onset or familial lobular breast cancers. J Med Genet. 2011;48:64–8.

46. Seal S, Thompson D, Renwick A, Elliott A, Kelly P, Barfoot R, et al. Truncating mutations in the Fanconi anemia J gene BRIP1 are low-penetrance breast cancer susceptibility alleles. Nat Genet. 2006;38:1239–41.

47. Seminog OO, Goldacre MJ. Age-specific risk of breast cancer in woman with neurofibromatosis type 1. BJC. 2015;112:1546–8.

48. Sharif S, Moran A, Huson SM, Iddenden R, Shenton A, Howard E, et al. Women with neurofibromatosis 1 are at a moderately increased risk of developing breast cancer and should be considered for early screening. J Med Genet. 2007;44:481–4.

49. Sokolenko AP, Preobrazhenskaya EV, Aleksakhina SN, Iyevleva AG, Mitiushkina NV, Zaitseva OA, et al. Candidate gene analysis of BRCA1/2 mutation-negative high-risk Russian breast cancer patients. Cancer Lett. 2015;359:259–61.

50. Steffen J, Nowakowska D, Niwinska A, Czapczak D, Kluska A, Piatkowska M, Wisniewska M, et al. Germline mutations 657del5 of the NBS1 gene contribute significantly to the incidence of breast cancer in Central Poland. Int J Can. 2006;119:472–5.

51. Swift M, Morrell D, Cromartie E, Chamberlin AR, Skolnick MH, Bishop DT. The incidence and gene frequency of ataxia-telangiectasia in the United States. Am J Hum Genet. 1986;39:573–83.

52. Tan MH, Mester J, Peterson C, Yang Y, Chen JL, Rybicki LA, et al. A clinical scoring system for selection of patients for PTEN mutation testing is proposed on the Basis of a Prospective Study of 3042 probands. Am J Hum Genet. 2011;88:42–56.

53. Tan MH, Mester JL, Ngeow J, Rybicki LA, Orloff MS, Eng C. Lifetime cancer risks in individuals with germline PTEN mutations. Clin Cancer Res. 2012;18:400–7.

54. Thai TH, Du F, Tsan JT, Jin Y, Phung A, Spillman MA, et al. Mutations in the BRCA1-associated RING domain (BARD1) gene in primary breast, ovarian and uterine cancers. Hum Mol Genet. 1998;7:195–202.

55. Tommiska J, Seal S, Renwick A, Barfoot R, Baskcomb L, Jayatilake H, et al. Evaluation of RAD50 in familial breast cancer predisposition. Int J Can. 2006;118:2911–6.

56. Varley JM. Germline TP53 mutations and Li-Fraumeni syndrome. Hum Mutat. 2003;21:313–20.

57. Varon R, Demuth I, Digweed M. Nijmegen breakage syndrome. 17 May 1999 [Updated 8 May 2014]. In: Pagon RA, Adam MP, Ardinger HH, et al., editors. GeneReviews® [Internet]. Seattle: University of Washington; 1993–2015. Available from: http://www.ncbi.nlm.nih.gov/books/NBK1176/.

58. Wang X, Levin AM, Smolinski SE, Vigneau FD, Levin NK, Tainsky MA. Breast cancer and other neoplasms in women with neurofibromatosis type1: a retrospective review of cases in the Detroit metropolitan area. Am Med Genet A. 2012;158A:3061–4.

59. Weischer M, Bojesen SE, Ellervik C, Tybjærg-Hansen A, Nordestgaard BG. CHEK2*1100decC Genotyping for clinical assessment of breast cancer risk: meta-analyses of 26,000 patient cases and 27,000 controls. J Clini Oncolo. 2008;26:542–8.

60. Whittemore AS, Gong G, John EM, McGuire V, Li VP, Ostrow KL, et al. Prevalence of BRCA1 mutation carriers among U.S. Non-Hispanic Whites. Cancer Epidemiol Biomarkers Prev. 2004;13:2078–83.

61. Wong MW, Nordfors C, Mossman D, Pecenpetelovska G, Avery-Kiejda A, Talseth-Palmer B, et al. BRIP1, PALB2, and RAD51C mutation analysis reveals their relative importance as genetic susceptibility factors for breast cancer. Breast Cancer Res Treat. 2011;127:853–9.
62. Xie ZM, Li LS, Laquet C, Penault-Llorca F, Uhrhammer N, Xie XM, et al. Germline mutations of the E-cadherin gene in families with inherited invasive lobular breast carcinoma but no diffuse gastric cancer. Cancer. 2011;117:3112–7.

Online Resources

American Board of Medical Genetics and Genomics. www.acmg.org.
GeneReviews. www.ncbi.nlm.nih.gov/books/NBK1116/.
National Society of Genetic Counselors. www.nsgc.org.
National Human Genome Research Institute. www.genome.gov.

Chapter 5
BRCA Patient Population

Alain Mina and Lida A. Mina

5.1 Hereditary Breast Cancer

Less than 10 % of breast cancers are due to hereditary triggers. The majority are hereditary mutations in single, dominant genes although more recent hypotheses are suggesting the implication of yet unidentified genes in a larger proportion of the sporadic cluster of breast cancers.

The type of cancer, early age of onset, and the number of generations in a particular family affected by it are all evidences of a potential hereditary trigger to breast cancer [1]. Ever since the late 1980s, numerous genes have been identified that conferred a certain susceptibility to its carrier through various mechanisms, be it via the acquisition of function or the lack of. The former were called proto-oncogenes: These are normally regulators of cellular division and differentiation. Once altered by mutations, translocations, or epigenetic mechanisms, they become "oncogenes" and are associated with excessively high levels of expression of "oncoproteins" rendering cells insensitive to apoptosis-inducing signals. Uncontrolled and unchecked proliferation ensues [2]. The latter are tumor suppressor genes. These are associated with dampening effects on cell cycle progression [3] and, unlike oncogenes, follow the two-hit hypothesis, meaning they require both alleles to be lost for oncogenesis to take place.

A. Mina, MD
Resident Physician, Kansas University Medical Center, Kansas City, KS, USA

L.A. Mina, MD (✉)
Director of the Catherine Peachy Breast Cancer Prevention Program,
Assistant Professor of Clinical Medicine, IU Simon Cancer Center,
Indiana University School of Medicine, Indianapolis, IN, USA
e-mail: lmina@iu.edu

© Springer International Publishing Switzerland 2016
L.A. Mina et al. (eds.), *Breast Cancer Prevention and Treatment*,
DOI 10.1007/978-3-319-19437-0_5

5.2   BRCA1 and BRCA2

The most clinically relevant genes associated with breast cancer are the BRCA1 and BRCA2 genes, on chromosomes 17q21 and 13q12, respectively. Mutations in these genes are germ line, transferred in an autosomal dominant fashion, and are exceptionally penetrant [4]. These confer to their carriers a breast cancer risk up to 30 times as high as that of the general population [5]. As mentioned earlier, an early age of onset (typically less than 50) coupled with multiple cases of breast cancer within the same family, male breast cancer, as well as the bilateral breast cancer all raises suspicion into a hereditary form of the malignancy [6]. BRCA1 and BRCA2 gene mutations are rare in the general population (1 of 400 persons), but their prevalence is higher in certain subpopulations such as the Ashkenazi Jewish population where, strikingly, 1 of 40 persons carry the mutations likely accounted for by a pronounced founder's effect which makes genetic testing among these groups more targeted [1].

BRCA1 and BRCA2 generate very large proteins (2843 and 3418 amino acids, respectively), and although deleterious missense mutations have been described, like most tumor suppressor genes, mutations resulting in a truncated protein have been found culprit [6]. Following their introduction in 1994 by Myriad Genetics, their clinical implications were instantly understood, and they have since been thoroughly studied. Their patterns of expression and localization have been described and found to be shared with RAD51, a mammalian homologue of RecA, an *Escherichia coli* (*E. coli*) protein essential for repair of double-stranded DNA breaks. Both BRCA proteins have been reported to bind and interact with RAD51, and although their role has not been entirely elucidated, it appears that these proteins are essential for a proper cellular response to DNA damage and the maintenance of chromosomal integrity [7].

The markedly increased susceptibility to breast cancers in carriers of BRCA mutations has been well established, but the magnitude of the associated risk has been inconsistently quantified largely due to the discrepancies in breast cancer risk factors among the different study populations. Reliable estimates of the cancer risk associated with BRCA mutations are however crucial for proper planning and individualization of management. A meta-analysis clustering data from ten studies in 2007 established a cumulative risk of breast cancer at 70 years of age of 57 % (95% CI, 47–66 %) for BRCA1 and 49 % (95 % CI, 40–57 %) for BRCA2 mutation carriers. Same study found a cumulative risk of ovarian cancer of 40 % (95 % CI, 35–46 %) for BRCA1 mutation carriers and 18 % (95 % CI, 13–23 %) for BRCA2 mutation carriers at 70 years of age [8].

The characterization of the role of BRCA1 and BRCA2 gene mutations in the pathogenesis of breast cancer has had a huge effect on management of carrier cases and clinical outcome. And with the advances in gene sequencing, particularly next-generation sequencing, this discovery paved the way for a novel strategy of management: The identification of more genes that would be implied in tumorigenesis and would allow a somewhat reliable prediction of outcome. Targeted DNA amplification coupled with next-generation sequencing leads to the identification of several suscepti-bility genes with moderate and high correlation with cancer risk such as ATM, RAD50, CHEK2, and TP53 with associated cancer risks of 5 %, 3 %, 2 %, and 1 %, respec-tively. Other identified mutations such as MAP3K1, ZNF217, ERBB2, and RAD51B were found to predict a markedly increased HER2 expression [9]. The implications of similar clusters of genes when put together in a clinical context are limitless.

Inherited susceptibility to breast malignancy has not only been linked to certain genetic variants of the BRCA genes but to several well-known syndromes, for instance, a germ line mutation in the tumor suppressor gene TP53 is associated with Li-Fraumeni syndrome: carriers are at risk of a number of primary cancers beginning in childhood such as sarcomas (of bone and soft tissue), brain tumors, and leukemias. The lifetime cancer risk for females with Li-Fraumeni syndrome is close to a 100 %, and one of the most commonly seen malignancy is actually premenopausal breast cancer with a mean age of onset of less than 35 [10, 11].

Another dominantly inherited syndrome largely associated with breast cancer is the Peutz-Jeghers syndrome (PJS). PJS is a rare genetic disease associated with a number of benign and malignant tumors of several organ systems [12]. Germ line mutations in the serine/threonine kinase 11 genes located on chromosome 19p were found culprit. The lifetime cumulative cancer risk of breast cancer in women with mutated STK11 is close to 55 % with a mean age of onset of only 37 [13, 14].

Cowden syndrome (also PTEN hamartoma syndrome) is another inherited syndrome that accounts for an increased susceptibility to breast malignancy and a much earlier age of onset. Mutations in PTEN (phosphatase and tensin homologue), a tumor suppressor gene linked to Cowden syndrome, account for a wide spectrum of malignancies ranging from mucocutaneous and hamartomatous tumors to solid tumors of the uterus, thyroid, and kidneys [15, 16]. In a prospective study of more than 3300 individuals with established Cowden syndrome diagnoses, the absolute lifetime risk of breast cancer was found to be 85.2 %, most at a premenopausal age and 50 % by the age of 50 [17]. And so it seems that the aforementioned strategy of personalizing management through a thorough investigation of each patient's clinical context, risk factors, and genetic susceptibilities is not only limited to the BRCA genes but to a wide spectrum of genetic variants accounting for different presentations, different malignancies, and different syndromes.

5.3   Male Breast Cancer

Male carriers are also at an increased risk of breast cancer though to a lesser degree than the female population, and susceptibility seems to be more pronounced in BRCA2 carriers as compared to BRCA1 carriers. The lifetime risk of breast malignancy is approximately 6 % in male carriers of the BRCA2 mutation as compared to 1 % in male carriers of the BRCA1 mutation and 0.1 % in the general population [18].

Hereditary predisposition to breast cancer in men, although seemingly compara-ble in essence to that of women in terms of the nature of the different genetic variants and syndromes, is much different in terms of the degree of penetrance and the quantitative risk each hereditary trait carries. For instance, as mentioned earlier, although male BRCA gene mutation carriers do have a much higher breast cancer susceptibility than those of the general population, the association between genetic trait and clinical outcome is far less pronounced than the association of BRCA mutations with breast cancer in women. Similarly, mutations in the PTEN tumor suppressor genes accounting for Cowden syndrome have been linked to an increase in breast cancer risk among the male population. Men with TP53 mutations and the ensuing Li-Fraumeni syndrome have also been linked to a significant increase in lifetime breast cancer risk. But the numbers are far from those seen within the female population. In fact, the absolute risk of breast cancer in males remains quite low when compared to the general population, and so it is not common practice to advise screening via imaging or prophylactic procedures (such mastectomies) in this subpopulation regardless of the genetic trait that a man may carry.

5.4 BRCA and Other Malignancies

Though germ line BRCA mutations are notorious for their markedly increased breast and ovarian cancer risks, cancers elsewhere have also been a major concern. In a cohort study of approximately 12 000 individuals from 700 families harboring the BRCA1 mutation, chosen from 30 sites across Europe and North America, carriers of the mutation were found to be at a markedly increased risk for several other malignancies. For instance, when compared to the cancer incidence rates of the general population, risk of pancreatic cancer and cancers of the uterine body and cervix were significantly more pronounced in the former group with relative risks of 2.26, 2.65, and 3.72 for pancreatic, uterine body, and cervix malignancies, respectively [19].

Likewise, BRCA2 mutation carriers have been found susceptible to a wide spectrum of malignancies not limited to breast or ovarian. A study performed on 173 families, chosen across Europe and North America, showed a statistically significant increase in GI and skin cancer risks in carriers of the BRCA2 mutation. Gallbladder and bile duct cancer risks were the most prominent in this subpopulation with an estimated relative risk of 4.97 (95 % CI = 1.50–16.52), followed by prostate cancer with an estimated RR of 4.65 (95 % CI = 3.48–6.22), pancreatic with 3.51 (95 % CI = 1.87–6.58), stomach with 2.59 (95 % CI = 1.46–4.61), and melanomas with 2.58 (95 % CI = 1.28–5.17). The relative risk of prostate cancer for men under the age of 65 was found to be a staggering 7.33 (95 % CI = 4.66–11.52) [4, 20], and almost 15 years following that study, guidelines have emerged promoting the screening for prostate malignancy in all male carriers of the BRCA mutations, beginning at 40 years of age [21]. And so it is a must that physicians keep in mind the versatility of the malignancies at risk whenever managing or following up with carriers of the BRCA mutations irrespective of gender or cancer status.

As mentioned earlier, it has become common knowledge that a positive BRCA mutation status is highly associated with breast and ovarian cancers. More so,

BRCA mutations are accountable for a significantly higher lifetime risk of other primary cancers in their carriers such as the pancreas, uterus, prostate, and biliary tract. Other worthwhile observations that are yet to be as conclusively elucidated are those that associate particular phenotypic, molecular, and imaging characteristics of breast cancer with the BRCA mutation status to the point where, as we will see later on, a simple finding on MRI could justify a genetic testing for a BRCA mutation.

5.5   BRCA Testing

In the United States and much of the European countries, BRCA testing is only warranted (and more importantly covered) if the risk of detecting a BRCA mutation is more than 10 % (American Society of Clinical Oncology, 2003). However, it seems that with the growing understanding of the strength of the association between certain phenotypic and radiologic findings with BRCA status, efforts will move into recommending genetic testing not only in those with a suggestive family history but a suggestive phenotypic, pathological, and even MRI findings.

BRCA1 mutation carriers are more likely to have a triple-negative disease, i.e., a cancer that does not express the estrogen (ER), the progesterone (PR), or the human epidermal growth factor receptors (HER2). Triple-negative disease has its own phenotypic implications, such as its association with an earlier onset, a higher mitotic index, a less favorable histological grade, a higher tendency for distance spread, and an overall decreased survival [22–24]. Similarly, BRCA1 mutation carriers with the triple-negative disease seem to have a more aggressive tumor with a less favorable nuclear grade [22]. Despite the aforementioned correlation between BRCA mutation status and triple-negative disease (TND), not all women with TND qualify to genetic testing. In fact, testing is currently dictated by an individual's family history, age of onset, and rarely, as mentioned earlier, ethnicity (as with the Ashkenazi Jews) [25]. Pathology has never been a strong enough criterion for genetic testing, but this strong association between TND and BRCA mutation has led to a school of thought that promotes genetic testing in women with TND regardless of their age or family history. Some studies have established a likelihood of 20 % of carrying a BRCA mutation in women with triple-negative breast cancer, and that the triple-negative phenotype ought to be added to the list of criteria with absolute indication for genetic testing. The NCCN guidelines currently added triple-negative cancer in women below the age of 60 as an indication for BRCA testing.

5.6   BRCA Screening and Imaging

Screening of women is no longer limited to mammography. Numerous studies have established, without a doubt, a superior role for magnetic resonance imaging (MRI) over ultrasound or mammography in the screening of women with high risk for breast malignancy in terms of their family history and genetic testing. A systematic review of these studies has found a much lower sensitivity for mammography (13–40 %) when compared to MRI (71–100 %) [26]. Another review has shown that mammography, when combined to MRI, yielded the most optimal imaging results and the highest benefit for women with high-risk family history or genetic testing [27]. Since then, guidelines have emerged from the American Cancer Society and the United Kingdom that recommend yearly breast MRIs, with or without mammography for women with known BRCA mutation carrier status or an unknown carrier status but a first-degree relative that is positive for BRCA1 or BRCA2 mutation [28]. But could the role of MRI exceed that of simple screening and carry more diagnostic implications? Triple-negative disease has been associated with a characteristic oval shape, smooth margins, and rim enhancement on MRI [29]. Rim enhancement has long been established as a reliable predictor of an unfavorable disease course due to its association with a higher and more aggressive tumor grade [30]. Since it has been established that BRCA1 mutations are in fact highly associated with triple-negative disease and a higher nuclear grade with a less favorable course, MRI findings such as the smooth shape and rim enhancement could in fact account for a BRCA-positive disease, but whether a suspicious lesion with the above features on MRI warrants genetic testing is yet to be determined [31]. A 2009 review of MRI imaging results in female carriers of the BRCA1 and BRCA2 mutations showed that the latter had "poorly defined, with irregular or spiculated margins and ringlike enhancement patterns," and no noteworthy pathological differences on MRI were seen between the different genetic subtypes [31, 32].

5.7 Surgical Approach in BRCA

As previously mentioned, the majority of patients with a hereditary predisposition to breast or ovarian cancers are carriers of either of the BRCA gene mutations. These will not only carry marked susceptibilities to breast and ovarian cancers but a wide variety of oncological malignancies of the fallopian tubes, prostate, and pancreas. In what follows, we will be discussing the proper and comprehensive management of BRCA1 and BRCA2 mutation carriers in women without a cancer diagnosis.

In patients without a cancer diagnosis, bilateral prophylactic mastectomies have been shown to be associated with up to 95 % reduction in risk of breast malignancy in BRCA mutation carriers, hence achieving a breast cancer risk that is similar and even lower than that of the general population [33, 34].

Similarly, bilateral prophylactic salpingo-oophorectomy (BSO) has been associated with a 90 % reduction in ovarian cancer risk; the remaining risk is that of primary peritoneal carcinomatosis, a pathologically indistinguishable entity from ovarian cancer [35]. Add to that an independent associated decrease in breast cancer risk estimated at 50 % and a breast cancer protection rate of 73 % in BRCA2 mutation carriers when performed premenopausally [35, 36]. But what about the surgically induced menopause in patients having undergone BSO? An instantaneous consequence of BSO in pre- and perimenopausal women is menopause and all its distresses, whether physical such as hot flashes, genital dryness, and sexual dysfunction or psychological such as anxiety, labile or depressed affect, decreased libido, etc. Consequently, many women will elect to use hormone replacement therapy (HRT) to ease the severity of these symptoms and improve quality of life, while others may refrain from doing so because of concerns about hormonal therapy increasing their breast cancer risk, especially given their younger age. Several studies have shown that HRT does not annul the beneficial effects of BSO with regard to breast malignancy risk, and that the use of HRT was not significantly associated with an independent increase in breast cancer risk in women having undergone BSO [37, 38].

For carriers of the BRCA gene mutations that have chosen not to undergo prophylactic surgeries, close cancer surveillance would be the second best option: These women should be educated about all the possible signs and symptoms of breast/ovarian cancers. Ovarian cancer screening should be considered through concurrent vaginal ultrasounds and CA 125 level measurements starting 30 years of age or up to 10 years before the earliest age of ovarian cancer diagnosis in the family. As for breast cancer surveillance, self-breast exams should be performed beginning at age 18 and clinical examination by a specialist at age 25, every 6–12 months. Annual mammography should also be performed starting at the age of 25 or individualized according to the earliest age of breast cancer diagnosis in the family according to the NCCN guidelines.

5.8 Chemoprevention in BRCA

As for tamoxifen use as a chemopreventive regimen in BRCA mutation carriers, some data is available that shows a breast cancer risk reduction of 62 % in female carriers of the BRCA2 mutation but not in BRCA1. This can be largely explained by the fact that the greatest benefit of tamoxifen is observed in estrogen-positive tumors, and BRCA2 mutations are more likely to coexist with an ER-positive status than BRCA1 [39].

Another similarity in management between patients with or without a history of cancer with a positive BRCA mutation status would be a significant impact on mortality and risk reduction with bilateral salpingo-oophorectomy, especially those in whom future childbearing is not a consideration. In 2561 patients with a previous breast cancer diagnosis, BSO leads to a significant reduction in all-cause mortality (HR 0.32, 95 % CI 0.26–0.39, $p < 0.001$), in both BRCA1 and BRCA2 mutation carriers [40].

Similarly, chemoprevention with tamoxifen leads to a reduction in incidence of contralateral breast malignancy in both BRCA1 and BRCA2 mutation carriers with a breast cancer diagnosis, and this effect was independent of the estrogen receptor status of the initial cancer [41].

5.9 In Summary

BRCA mutation carriers are at significant increase of multiple malignancies including breast cancer. The approach to their care should be tailored to early prevention as well as aggressive screening protocols to avoid any effect of the disease on their long-term survival. Further details will also be discussed at later chapters.

References

1. Foulkes WD. Inherited susceptibility to common cancers. N Engl J Med. 2008;359(20): 2143–53.
2. Croce CM. Oncogenes and cancer. N Engl J Med. 2008;358(5):502–11.
3. Sherr CJ. Principles of tumor suppression. Cell. 2004;116(2):235–46.
4. Breast Cancer Linkage, C. Cancer risks in BRCA2 mutation carriers. J Natl Cancer Inst. 1999;91(15):1310–6.
5. Antoniou A, et al. Average risks of breast and ovarian cancer associated with BRCA1 or BRCA2 mutations detected in case Series unselected for family history: a combined analysis of 22 studies. Am J Hum Genet. 2003;72(5):1117–30.
6. Foulkes WD, Shuen AY. In brief: BRCA1 and BRCA2. J Pathol. 2013;230(4):347–9.
7. Venkitaraman AR. Functions of BRCA1 and BRCA2 in the biological response to DNA damage. J Cell Sci. 2001;114(Pt 20):3591–8.
8. Chen S, Parmigiani G. Meta-analysis of BRCA1 and BRCA2 penetrance. J Clin Oncol. 2007;25(11):1329–33.
9. Aloraifi F, et al. Detection of novel germline mutations for breast cancer in non-BRCA1/2 families. FEBS J. 2015;282(17):3424–37.
10. Malkin D. Li-fraumeni syndrome. Genes Cancer. 2011;2(4):475–84.
11. Olivier M, et al. Li-Fraumeni and related syndromes: correlation between tumor type, family structure, and TP53 genotype. Cancer Res. 2003;63(20):6643–50.
12. Hemminki A, et al. A serine/threonine kinase gene defective in Peutz-Jeghers syndrome. Duodecim. 1998;114(7):667–8.
13. Giardiello FM, et al. Very high risk of cancer in familial Peutz-Jeghers syndrome. Gastroenterology. 2000;119(6):1447–53.
14. Beggs AD, et al. Peutz-Jeghers syndrome: a systematic review and recommendations for management. Gut. 2010;59(7):975–86.
15. Pilarski R, et al. Cowden syndrome and the PTEN hamartoma tumor syndrome: systematic review and revised diagnostic criteria. J Natl Cancer Inst. 2013;105(21):1607–16.
16. Eng C. PTEN hamartoma tumor syndrome (PHTS). In: Pagon RA et al., editors. GeneReviews(R). Seattle: University of Washington; 1993.
17. Tan MH, et al. Lifetime cancer risks in individuals with germline PTEN mutations. Clin Cancer Res. 2012;18(2):400–7.
18. Liede A, Karlan BY, Narod SA. Cancer risks for male carriers of germline mutations in BRCA1 or BRCA2: a review of the literature. J Clin Oncol. 2004;22(4):735–42.
19. Thompson D, Easton DF, Breast Cancer C. Linkage, cancer incidence in BRCA1 mutation carriers. J Natl Cancer Inst. 2002;94(18):1358–65.
20. Mavaddat N, et al. Cancer risks for BRCA1 and BRCA2 mutation carriers: results from prospective analysis of EMBRACE. J Natl Cancer Inst. 2013;105(11):812–22.
21. Mitra AV, et al. Targeted prostate cancer screening in men with mutations in BRCA1 and BRCA2 detects aggressive prostate cancer: preliminary analysis of the results of the IMPACT study. BJU Int. 2011;107(1):28–39.

22. Atchley DP, et al. Clinical and pathologic characteristics of patients with BRCA-positive and BRCA-negative breast cancer. J Clin Oncol. 2008;26(26):4282–8.
23. Rakha EA, Reis-Filho JS, Ellis IO. Basal-like breast cancer: a critical review. J Clin Oncol. 2008;26(15):2568–81.
24. Dent R, et al. Triple-negative breast cancer: clinical features and patterns of recurrence. Clin Cancer Res. 2007;13(15 Pt 1):4429–34.
25. Wong-Brown MW, et al. Prevalence of BRCA1 and BRCA2 germline mutations in patients with triple-negative breast cancer. Breast Cancer Res Treat. 2015;150(1):71–80.
26. Elmore JG, et al. Screening for breast cancer. JAMA. 2005;293(10):1245–56.
27. Narod SA. Screening of women at high risk for breast cancer. Prev Med. 2011;53(3):127–30.
28. Chiarelli AM, et al. Effectiveness of screening with annual magnetic resonance imaging and mammography: results of the initial screen from the ontario high risk breast screening program. J Clin Oncol. 2014;32(21):2224–30.
29. Uematsu T, Kasami M, Yuen S. Triple-negative breast cancer: correlation between MR imaging and pathologic findings. Radiology. 2009;250(3):638–47.
30. Lee SH, et al. Correlation between high resolution dynamic MR features and prognostic factors in breast cancer. Korean J Radiol. 2008;9(1):10–8.
31. Noh JM, et al. Association between BRCA mutation status, pathological findings, and magnetic resonance imaging features in patients with breast cancer at risk for the mutation. J Breast Cancer. 2013;16(3):308–14.
32. Gilbert FJ, et al. Cancers in BRCA1 and BRCA2 carriers and in women at high risk for breast cancer: MR imaging and mammographic features. Radiology. 2009;252(2):358–68.
33. Hollingsworth AB, et al. Current comprehensive assessment and management of women at increased risk for breast cancer. Am J Surg. 2004;187(3):349–62.
34. Rebbeck TR, et al. Bilateral prophylactic mastectomy reduces breast cancer risk in BRCA1 and BRCA2 mutation carriers: the PROSE Study Group. J Clin Oncol. 2004;22(6):1055–62.
35. Kauff ND, et al. Risk-reducing salpingo-oophorectomy for the prevention of BRCA1- and BRCA2-associated breast and gynecologic cancer: a multicenter, prospective study. J Clin Oncol. 2008;26(8):1331–7.
36. Pruthi S, Gostout BS, Lindor NM. Identification and management of women with BRCA mutations or hereditary predisposition for breast and ovarian cancer. Mayo Clin Proc. 2010;85(12):1111–20.
37. Rebbeck TR, et al. Effect of short-term hormone replacement therapy on breast cancer risk reduction after bilateral prophylactic oophorectomy in BRCA1 and BRCA2 mutation carriers: the PROSE Study Group. J Clin Oncol. 2005;23(31):7804–10.
38. Rebbeck TR, et al. Breast cancer risk after bilateral prophylactic oophorectomy in BRCA1 mutation carriers. J Natl Cancer Inst. 1999;91(17):1475–9.
39. King MC, et al. Tamoxifen and breast cancer incidence among women with inherited mutations in BRCA1 and BRCA2: National Surgical Adjuvant Breast and Bowel Project (NSABP-P1) Breast Cancer Prevention Trial. JAMA. 2001;286(18):2251–6.
40. Finch AP, et al. Impact of oophorectomy on cancer incidence and mortality in women with a BRCA1 or BRCA2 mutation. J Clin Oncol. 2014;32(15):1547–53.
41. Gronwald J, et al. Tamoxifen and contralateral breast cancer in BRCA1 and BRCA2 carriers: an update. Int J Cancer. 2006;118(9):2281–4.

Chapter 6
Proliferative Breast Disease

Kandice K. Ludwig

6.1 Introduction

The term benign breast disease (BBD) encompasses a group of histologically diverse pathologic diagnoses. It is quite common, although data regarding the prevalence is limited. Autopsy data demonstrates significant variation in prevalence rates, ranging from 5 to 60 %. It is estimated that approximately 50 % of women will develop some sort of BBD after age 20 [1].

In the current era of breast imaging with high-resolution digital mammography, most patients with BBD are asymptomatic and present with abnormal findings on imaging prompting additional workup. A percentage of patients will present with clinical symptoms, such as a palpable mass or nipple discharge. Once diagnostic imaging is performed and a lesion identified, it is standard of care to establish the diagnosis using percutaneous core needle biopsy (CNB) [2].

Histologically, BBD can be subdivided into three categories, depending on the degree of epithelial proliferation. Dupont and Page established criteria for classification of these lesions in 1985, after reviewing biopsy slides from 3000 women in the Nashville Cohort. *Nonproliferative lesions* include cysts, papillary apocrine change, epithelial-related calcifications, and usual hyperplasia. Lesions classified as *proliferative* include florid ductal hyperplasia, intraductal papillomas, sclerosing adenosis, radial scars, and fibroadenomas. *Atypical ductal and lobular hyperplasias* are proliferative lesions that possess some but not all of the features of carcinoma in situ [3].

It has been hypothesized that some of these lesions are stages within the histologic continuum leading to invasive breast cancer. Carefully performed epidemiologic studies of large cohorts of women have contributed to our ability to estimate risk of

K.K. Ludwig, MD
Department of Surgery, Indiana University School of Medicine, Indianapolis, IN, USA
e-mail: kaludwig@iupui.edu

© Springer International Publishing Switzerland 2016   59
L.A. Mina et al. (eds.), *Breast Cancer Prevention and Treatment*,
DOI 10.1007/978-3-319-19437-0_6

Table 6.1 Relative risk of breast cancer in women with benign breast disease

Author	Type of study	Nonproliferative (95 % CI)	Proliferative disease (95 % CI)	Atypical hyperplasia (95 % CI)
Dupont, Page, 1985 [3]	Case–cohort	Reference group	1.9 (1.2–2.9)	5.3 (3.1–8.8)
Collins, 2007 [4]	Case–control	Reference group	1.52 (1.2–2.0)	4.11 (2.9–5.8)
Zhou, 2011 [5]	Meta-analysis	Reference group	1.44 (1.28–1.63)	2.81 (1.91–4.12)
Dyrstad, 2015 [6]	Meta-analysis	1.2 (0.94–1.47)	1.76 (1.58–1.95)	3.93 (3.24–4.76)

breast cancer development associated with these lesions. These studies have confirmed that women whose biopsies demonstrate nonproliferative changes only harbor no increase in breast cancer risk when compared to the average population [3]. Women with proliferative epithelial changes are at increased risk of breast cancer, especially when associated with atypia (Table 6.1) [3–6]. As reported by a recent meta-analysis of 34 studies in women with benign breast disease, women with proliferative changes were 1.8 times more likely to develop breast cancer, and women with atypical hyperplasia had approximately four times higher risk [6].

Once the diagnosis of a proliferative lesion is made on CNB, the clinician should first address whether there exists a need for surgical excision to obtain more tissue for evaluation. Additionally, the patient should be stratified regarding her risk of breast cancer. Discussions regarding risk stratification include potential enhanced surveillance and risk reduction.

Surveys polling both radiologists and practicing surgeons have shown lack of consensus in recommendations regarding management of some of these proliferative lesions [7]. This is likely secondary to lack of randomized prospective data. Overtreatment can result in unnecessary procedures, cost, and potential complications for the patient, while undertreatment could possibly miss a breast cancer. The purpose of this chapter is to review the common proliferative breast conditions, focusing on initial management (including need for surgical excision) and long-term risk of breast cancer development.

6.2 Flat Epithelial Atypia

Flat epithelial atypia (FEA) is a benign proliferative lesion, characterized by alteration of the native epithelium within the terminal ductal–lobular unit [8, 9]. Affected ducts are often dilated and contain intraluminal microcalcifications; the association of FEA with mammographic calcifications is well documented in the literature [10]. There has been an increase in frequency of this lesion with enhanced use of mammography [8]. The true incidence is unknown, as there has been variance in the pathologic definition. It was previously known as "clinging carcinoma" or "columnar cell change with atypia." FEA has been reported within 2.4–3.7 % of core biopsy specimens and 0.1 % of reduction mammoplasty specimens [8, 9, 11].

The clinical significance of FEA is under debate; there is controversy as to whether the presence of FEA on core biopsy mandates surgical excision and whether patients with FEA have an increased risk of future breast cancer development. Historically most patients diagnosed by CNB were offered excision to evaluate for possible coexisting carcinoma. A meta-analysis of 22 studies looking at the presence of coexisting carcinoma after excisional biopsy for FEA alone demonstrated significant heterogeneity, ranging from 0 to 67 %. The pooled underestimation rate was 17 % with 57 of 389 patients exhibiting cancer at excision, prompting the authors to recommend surgical excision [12]. Calhoun and colleagues retrospectively reviewed 210 core biopsies demonstrating FEA with radiographic–pathologic concordance and subsequent surgical excision. In their series of 73 patients with pure FEA (with no additional lesions), only five were upgraded (7 %). Interestingly, in patients who underwent biopsies for calcifications, complete removal of the calcifications was associated with a 0 % upgrade rate [10].

FEA may be a surface manifestation of underlying architectural atypia. A significant portion of patients with FEA on core biopsy will have associated atypical hyperplasia. If both FEA and atypical hyperplasia are present on CNB, the risk of upgrade to malignancy on excision increases to 26 % [12]. Up to 46 % of patients with pure FEA on core biopsy will demonstrate the presence of atypia on excisional biopsy [8, 9]. While these patients with associated atypia are not upgraded to a cancer diagnosis, this information may be important for risk stratification [10].

Few studies contain data evaluating patients with pure FEA in the absence of atypical hyperplasia. Furthermore, almost all lack data regarding radiographic–pathologic correlation. Both can result in an increase of coexisting carcinomas seen at surgical excision. The authors of the meta-analysis concluded that surgical excision should be considered in patients with FEA [12]. Other authors suggest that in patients with concordance of pathology and mammographic findings, one could consider observation with close surveillance in lieu of surgical excision, provided the majority of the calcifications were removed with CNB [10]. Uzoaru reported no malignancies after mean 5-year follow-up in 33 women with pure FEA on CNB without subsequent surgical excision [9]. Decisions regarding surgical excision should be individualized based on the patient's presentation, radiographic–pathologic concordance, and other risk factors.

6.2.1 Future Cancer Risk

Molecular analysis has demonstrated striking similarities in loss of heterozygosity between FEA and ductal carcinoma in situ (DCIS)/invasive carcinoma, leading to concern regarding risk of subsequent development of breast cancer [13]. However, Said and colleagues demonstrated the presence of FEA alone does not appear to be associated with an independent rise in breast cancer risk. Using the Mayo Benign Breast Disease Cohort, they reported a 6.7 % risk of subsequent breast cancer after median follow-up of 16.8 years. There was no increase in risk when accounting for other risk factors, such as family history, age at biopsy, and the presence of atypia [8].

6.3   Radial Scar/Complex Sclerosing Lesions

Radial scars (RS) and complex sclerosing lesions are benign lesions with features that mimic malignancy both on imaging and pathology. The mammographic appearance has been well documented, often presenting as architectural distortion with translucent center and elongated radial spiculations [14]. Histologically these lesions are infiltrative, characterized by a central area of necrotic material surrounded by a corona of epithelial proliferation (Fig. 6.1) [15]. Epithelial atypia is not characteristic, although they may coexist with other benign proliferative lesions and atypical hyperplasia [16]. Lesions less than 1 cm are classified as radial scars; lesions greater than 1 cm are complex sclerosing lesions. For simplicity, these lesions will be referred to as RS for the remainder of the section.

Radial scars are relatively common, as demonstrated by postmortem studies, with higher incidence in patients with proliferative breast disease or personal history of breast cancer [17]. Before the advent of mammographic screening, RS were mostly incidental findings on biopsy specimens removed for other reasons.

Prior to the advent of core biopsies, the mammographic findings consistent with RS were associated with a 20 % diagnosis of malignancy (range 10–41 %), leading to the practice of mandatory surgical excision. However, the data is not reflective of the current environment of improved mammographic technology. Furthermore, percutaneous core needle biopsy (CNB) is now the standard method to obtain histologic diagnosis of breast lesions, and current literature has shown reduction in upgrade rates with larger biopsy needle gauge and more extensive sampling. These issues have resulted in controversy whether patients diagnosed with RS by CNB can forego surgical excision. No prospective studies have been performed, and most data consists of retrospective analyses evaluating small institutional cohorts, with

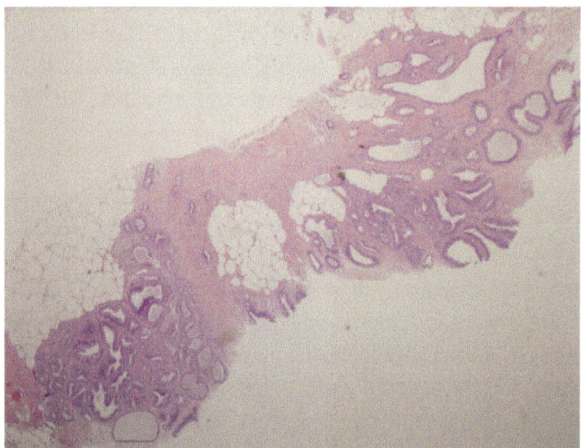

Fig. 6.1 Radial scar on core needle biopsy (magnification 40×). Central sclerotic area surrounded by benign epithelial structures. The radial orientation of the epithelium is somewhat visible

little information regarding radiographic–pathologic correlation. The presence of coexisting carcinoma on surgical excision in patients with RS on CNB is quite variable in the literature, ranging from 0 to 40 %. As reported by a meta-analysis of 20 studies evaluating 1255 lesions, upgrade to invasive carcinoma or DCIS was seen in 131 lesions (overall upgrade rate 10.4 %) [17].

There has been investigation to determine clinicopathologic factors that increase the risk of associated cancer with RS. Studies evaluating excisional biopsy for radiographic findings of RS suggest older age is associated with upgrade, as the presence of cancer with RS is extremely rare in patients less than 50 years of age [18, 19]. The presence of atypical hyperplasia within the lesion has been shown to increase the risk of upgrade significantly (27 % with atypia vs. 7.5 % without atypia) [17]. Furthermore, the histologic size of RS appears to be a significant risk factor on excisional biopsy, as lesions less than 1 cm exhibit significantly lower risk of associated cancers [18, 19].

However, in the current practice of CNB as initial diagnostic procedure, does the size of the RS correlate with risk of malignancy? Matrai and colleagues reviewed 66 patients with RS <5 mm on CNB and radiographic concordance and found no cancers on subsequent excision. They did note a 12 % upgrade to other high-risk lesions, such as atypical hyperplasia and lobular carcinoma in situ [20]. In a review of 38 patients with RS on CNB followed by surgical excision, Nassar et al. reported that radiographic size was an independent risk factor of upgrade, as no cancers were seen in lesions less than 1 cm [21].

Studies evaluating outcome for patients who do not undergo excisional biopsy for RS on CNB show minimal risk of cancer development, although the cohort sizes are small. Resetkova and colleagues followed 46 patients for median 29 months, with no cancers seen [22]. Brenner et al. noted similar findings in their cohort of 55 patients, with no patients developing cancer at median 38-month follow-up [23].

Significant variation still exists in current practice whether patients with RS on CNB should undergo surgical excision. In appropriate patients with small lesions, no associated atypia on CNB, and radiographic–pathologic correlation, one could consider imaging follow-up in lieu of surgical excision.

6.3.1 Future Cancer Risk

The similar appearance of epithelial elements in radial scars to that of carcinoma has prompted the hypothesis that RS may be an early precursor in the development of breast cancer. This has led to multiple studies investigating the long-term risk of breast cancer development in women with a diagnosis of RS, with conflicting results (Table 6.2). Jacobs and colleagues performed a case–control analysis of 99 women with RS as part of the Nurses' Health Study. With average follow-up of 12 years, they concluded that the presence of RS was an independent risk factor for development of breast cancer, with relative risk 1.8. This increase in risk was present regardless of any associated benign breast disease, such as proliferative changes

Table 6.2 Relative risk of breast cancer associated with radial scar

	Nurses' Health Study, 1999 [24]	Nashville Breast Cohort, 2006 [25]	Mayo Benign Breast Disease Cohort, 2008 [26]
Total women in cohort	1396	9556	9262
Number of women with RS	99	880	439
Follow-up length (years)	12	20.4	17
Relative risk of breast cancer	3.0 (95 % CI, 1.7–5.5)	1.82 years 1–10 (95 % CI, 1.2–2.7) 1.11 years 11+ (95 % CI, 0.77–1.6)	1.88 (95 % CI, 1.36–2.53)
Reference group	Nonproliferative disease	Women with nonproliferative disease, no RS	Iowa SEER registry
Type of study	Case–control	Retrospective cohort	Retrospective cohort

with and without atypia [24]. Similarly, a retrospective analysis of the Nashville Breast Cohort showed a slight increase in breast cancer risk in women with RS on excisional biopsy (RR 1.82) with the risk most significant within the first 10 years of follow-up. However, when accounting for other proliferative breast disease, the presence of RS did not add to baseline risk [25].

Furthermore, investigators at the Mayo Clinic performed a retrospective analysis of significance of RS in a cohort of 439 women with mean follow-up of 17 years; overall the relative risk was 1.88 for patients with RS, but was not an independent risk factor ($p=0.29$). The age of the patient, number of RS present on biopsy, and size of the RS also did not affect risk [26]. In all of the studies, subsequent cancers were seen within both breasts, questioning the role of these lesions as direct precursors rather than a response to a generalized phenomenon [24–26]. It is the current recommendation that the presence of RS should not be utilized as the sole criterion for counseling patients on enhanced surveillance or risk reduction strategies; this should be a comprehensive assessment based on the patient's other risk factors.

6.4 Papillary Lesions

Papillary lesions are a spectrum of intraductal proliferations characterized by varying grades of epithelial hyperplasia with an associated fibrovascular stalk (Fig. 6.2) [27]. They can range from simple benign intraductal papillomas to papillary adenocarcinomas. They are rare, accounting for 3.4 % of incidental lesions discovered in reduction mammoplasty specimens and 5 % of lesions on benign breast biopsy [11, 28]. Central lesions behind the nipple tend to be single and associated with symptoms of spontaneous nipple discharge; peripheral lesions tend to be smaller, can be multiple, and present with mass [29]. Radiographic findings include mass, calcifications, asymmetry, or distortion on mammography. Ultrasound

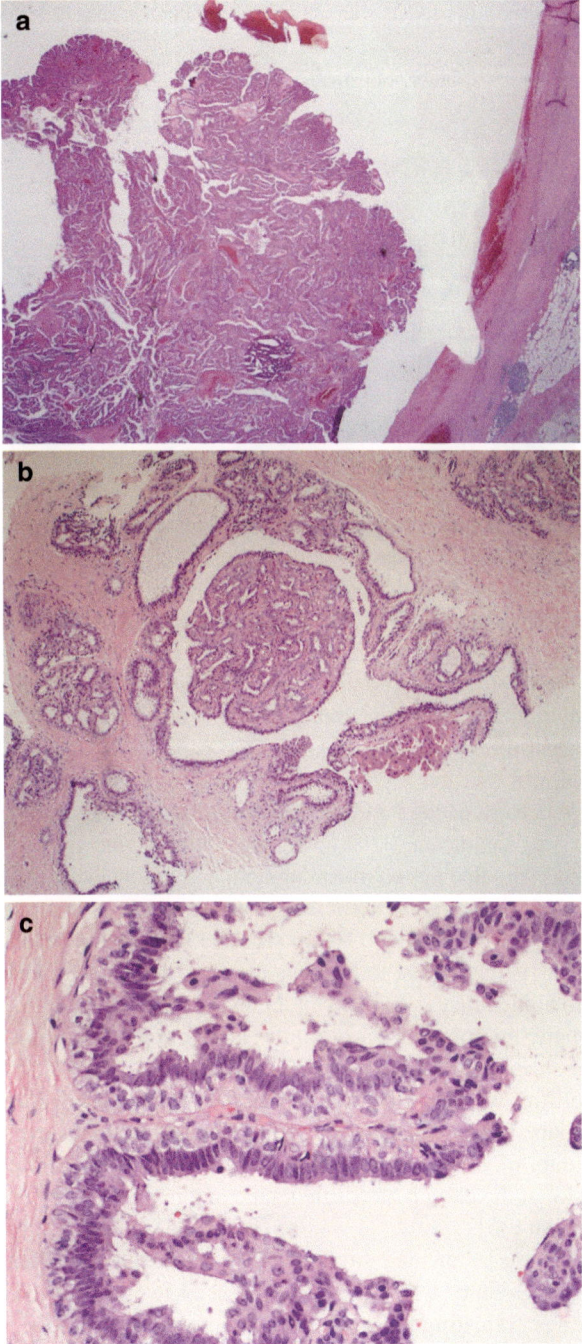

Fig. 6.2 (**a**) Large intraductal papilloma (magnification 100×). Papillary architecture is evident in the large papilloma even at this magnification. (**b**) Small intraductal papilloma (magnification 100×). (**c**) Intraductal papilloma (magnification 400×). High-power view of papillary architecture of a papilloma showing fibrovascular core and dual cell layer of the lining epithelium

Table 6.3 Risk of cancer in patients with intraductal papilloma managed with core biopsy alone and no surgical excision

Author	Number of patients	Follow-up (years)	Number of cancers seen (%)
Jaffer, 2013 [33]	23	3.0	0 (0)
Weisman, 2014 [34]	23	5.3	2 (8.7)
Wyss, 2014 [36]	156	3.5	2 (0.01)
Mosier, 2013 [37]	86	4.8	0 (0)
Swapp, 2013 [38]	100	3.0	0 (0)

may demonstrate intraductal mass with or without ductal ectasia. Galactography may show a well-defined filling defect with smooth borders [30].

Findings on imaging are not sufficient to accurately distinguish between benign and malignant lesions, so core needle biopsy (CNB) is the standard method of histologic diagnosis. In papillary lesions with atypia diagnosed by CNB, numerous studies have reported significant upgrade to malignancy at time of excision, with authors advocating routine surgical excision. However, there is little consensus regarding management of "pure" papillary lesions without atypia diagnosed by CNB, as studies report varying upgrade rates. However, these studies often include patients with variable presentations (symptomatic and asymptomatic, with and without associated atypia) that make conclusions difficult. There is often no data regarding radiographic concordance, and definitions vary regarding what is considered an upgrade (atypia vs. malignancy).

A meta-analysis of 34 studies evaluated 2236 papillary lesions diagnosed by CNB followed by surgical excision; a pooled 15.7 % upgrade to malignancy (range 3–42 %) was reported. When evaluating for clinicopathologic factors related to upgrade, the presence of atypia was significant (37 % malignancy with atypia vs. 7 % without atypia, $p=0.01$). Patients with findings on mammography were more likely to be upgraded [31].

The meta-analysis found no association with upgrade to malignancy with other factors, such as age of the patient, lesion size and location, or type/gauge of biopsy device [31]. This is in contrast to findings of other studies. McGhan et al. reported no upgrades to malignancy in women under 65 [32]. In two separate studies evaluating asymptomatic micropapillomas <2 mm, no upgrade to malignancy was seen at time of excision in 26 patients [33, 34]. Furthermore, Shamonki and colleagues sought to determine whether the amount of tissue sampled at CNB could distinguish a group of patients that could potentially be managed with observation alone; they noted the amount of tissue sampled at time of CNB was associated with upgrade and suggested that the choice of needle gauge and number of cores retrieved could benefit the patient [35].

As most of these lesions are small, it is hypothesized that often they are completely excised at time of CNB, avoiding the need for surgical excision in certain patients. In series evaluating follow-up for patients with intraductal papillomas with no associated atypia and concordant imaging, very few cancers are seen on follow-up without surgical excision. However, most of these studies have relatively short follow-up and small numbers of patients (Table 6.3) [33, 34, 36–38].

6.4.1 Future Cancer Risk

Once the decision has been made regarding need for excision, the clinician should also evaluate whether these patients should be considered for enhanced surveillance or risk reduction strategies. The largest study to evaluate subsequent cancer risk was reported by Lewis and colleagues using the Mayo Benign Breast Cohort. They retrospectively evaluated a cohort of 480 women with intraductal papillomas with mean follow-up of 14 years. They concluded that the presence of single benign papilloma did not independently raise the risk above that associated with proliferative breast disease, although the presence of atypia, especially with multiple papillomas, significantly increased subsequent breast cancer risk [29].

6.5 Atypical Ductal Hyperplasia

Atypical ductal hyperplasia (ADH) is a borderline lesion characterized by the presence of atypical cells within the terminal ductal–lobular unit (Fig. 6.3). It shares similar cytologic characteristics of ductal carcinoma in situ (DCIS), but lacks architectural features and differs in the amount of epithelial proliferation. Ninety percent of ADH shows high levels of expression to estrogen and progesterone receptors.

Atypical ductal hyperplasia is most commonly diagnosed on stereotactic core needle biopsy (CNB) targeting a cluster of mammographic microcalcifications. The presence of a mass lesion is the most common feature identified by ultrasound [39]. It is a rare condition, reportedly found in 1.8 % of breast reduction specimens and 8–10 % of breast biopsies [11, 40].

The standard initial management of a patient with ADH on CNB has been excisional biopsy to rule out underlying malignancy. Rates of incidence of

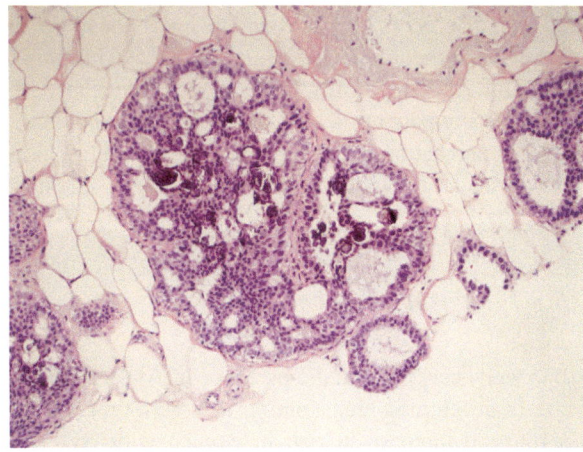

Fig. 6.3 Atypical ductal hyperplasia (magnification 200×). Cribriform intraductal proliferation with relatively round peripheral lumens. However, nuclei are small, hyperchromatic, and crowded at the center of the duct. Calcifications are present

malignancy at time of excisional biopsy in patients with ADH on CNB have ranged from 11 to 62 %. The distinction between ADH and DCIS is a quantitative one, based on the size of involvement and number of ducts involved, so additional tissue is often required. More recent series with current use of larger-gauge automated biopsy devices have demonstrated lower upstage rates. As a result, authors have sought to determine any clinical and pathologic factors would predict upgrade, hoping to select candidates that may be managed with imaging surveillance only.

As with most high-risk breast pathology, the data evaluating upstage rates of ADH and associated factors consists of retrospective analyses of single institutional series. There is significant selection bias and variation within the designs of these series, leading to inconsistent results. Factors including age of the patient, size of the lesion, number of cores removed, number of foci, micropapillary histology, and the presence of necrosis have all been investigated; some series report significant association with upgrade, while others do not. Some series have suggested reduced rates of cancer at time of excision with larger CNB devices; however, the risk of associated malignancy still ranges from 9 to 28 % with an 11-gauge vacuum-assisted device [41–43].

For patients presenting with microcalcifications as the targeted lesion, complete removal of the calcifications at time of CNB may be associated with reduced rates of upgrade at excisional biopsy, as shown by multiple series [43, 44]. These patients may be candidates for imaging surveillance rather than excisional biopsy. Villa et al. reported a series of 35 patients with no residual calcifications after CNB and imaging surveillance. At median follow-up of 53 months (range 6–72 months), only one woman developed cancer. This translated to a 1.6 % risk of malignancy in this selected group of patients, which they concluded would be within the accepted threshold for observation [44].

Some authors have investigated whether preoperative MRI could be used to identify features suggestive of upgrade at excision and could potentially spare patients an unnecessary surgical procedure. Small retrospective analyses suggest that MRI had high negative predictive value for high-risk lesions. However, in a meta-analysis of 16 studies evaluating MRI in this setting, no morphologic features were predictive of upgrade to malignancy [45]. These findings were confirmed in a prospective analysis of 16 patients with ADH, with false-negative rate of MRI at 10 %. The authors hypothesized this was due to the high upgrade rate (25 % in this cohort) and recommended against using MRI in this setting to avoid excision [46].

Future investigation will be needed, especially in the current era, to determine whether any patients with ADH would be candidates for imaging follow-up rather than excisional biopsy. At the current time, the standard recommendation would be for excision of all patients with ADH diagnosed on CNB.

6.5.1   Future Cancer Risk

It is well accepted that the presence of ADH within the breast increases a woman's risk of developing breast cancer in her lifetime. In 1985, Dupont and Page reported a fourfold increase in risk in women with ADH using data from the Nashville Cohort with 17-year median follow-up [3]. Additional studies have confirmed an increase in risk, although there is variation in the magnitude. Some studies include

ADH and atypical lobular hyperplasia together, while others evaluate them individually. A recent meta-analysis of six studies specifically evaluating future breast cancer risk with ADH demonstrating odds ratio (OR) of developing breast cancer was 3.3 (range 2.5–4.2). Mean time to development of cancer was 9.4 years for all patients in the meta-analysis [6].

Many authors have sought to determine factors that would further increase risk of developing breast cancer in these patients. Researchers at the Mayo Clinic noted younger age of biopsy was significant, although data from the Nurses' Health Study did not reveal a relationship with menopausal status [4, 47]. The race of the patient does not appear to be significant, as demonstrated by cohort of patients from the metropolitan Detroit area [1]. Whether the presence of a family history further increases risk is unclear. In the Nashville Cohort, a substantial increase in risk was reported in patients with atypical hyperplasia and a first-degree relative with breast cancer (OR 4.3 increased to 8.4) [3]. Newer studies do not confirm this finding. A meta-analysis of ten case–control studies of patients with high-risk lesions demonstrated no difference in risk for patients with atypical hyperplasia and family history [5]. The researchers at the Mayo Clinic in their report of long-term follow-up of 698 women with atypical hyperplasia also did not see any relationship with family history and future breast cancer development ($p=0.23$) [48].

There is still debate whether ADH is a direct precursor to breast cancer development or a marker of increased risk. Common genomic alterations and hormone receptor positivity have led some authors to suggest that atypical hyperplasia is a non-obligate precursor to low-grade DCIS and invasive cancers. If this were true, one would expect the preponderance of future cancers to develop within the ipsilateral breast, and cancers would develop within a relatively short interval. Multiple studies have shown only a 56 % risk of ipsilateral breast cancer risk with atypical hyperplasia [3, 4]. Hartmann et al. showed the risk of cancer development tends to favor the ipsilateral breast initially, but decreases with time to both breasts (82 % at 5 years, 58 % after 5 years) [48].

Regarding the interval from biopsy to cancer development, initial data noted the highest breast cancer risk within the first 10 years after biopsy (OR 9.8), with a significant drop after 10 years (OR 3.6) [3]. Other studies have reported the risk to persist with time. The Nurses' Health Study reported an increase in the odds ratio of developing breast cancer from 3.31 to 5.15 after 10 years [4]. Additionally, researchers at the Mayo Clinic reported a mean time of 10.3 years from biopsy to cancer development, with a persistent increase in risk, with 29 % incidence of breast cancer at 25-year follow-up. These results suggest that while some atypical lesions may be direct precursors, others are a marker of a microenvironment of increased risk [48].

6.6 Lobular Neoplasia

Lobular neoplasia encompasses a spectrum of atypical lesions characterized by distention of the terminal ductal–lobular unit by a population of discohesive cells. The distinction between atypical lobular neoplasia (ALH) and lobular carcinoma in situ (LCIS) is related to the amount of distention of the acinus; when there is greater

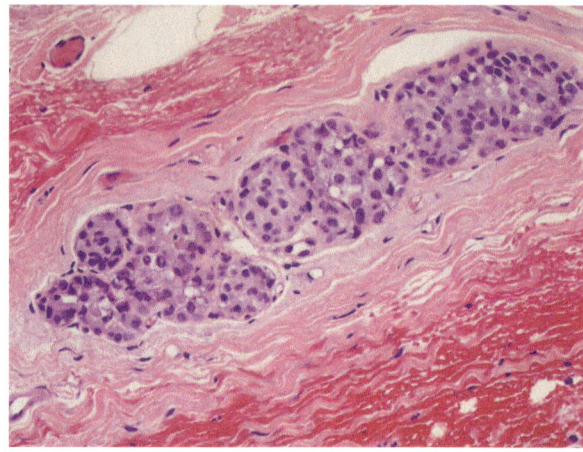

Fig. 6.4 Atypical lobular hyperplasia (magnification 400×). The normally visible acinar lumens from this small lobule are effaced. However, the individual acini are only minimally expanded and their borders are indistinct

than 50 % distention, it is considered LCIS (Figs. 6.4 and 6.5). Both ALH and LCIS characteristically show strong expression for estrogen receptors. Lack or downregulation of E-cadherin expression is seen in 95 % of patients with lobular neoplasia, leading to the characteristic appearance of discohesive cells [27, 49].

Lobular neoplasia is considered clinically occult, as most patients present with no changes on clinical exam or imaging. This was initially thought to be an incidental finding in breast biopsies performed for other reasons. However, in the current era of screening mammography, these lesions may be associated with calcifications in 65 % of patients, likely related to the presence of columnar cell change [49, 50]. The true incidence of these lesions is unknown; some suggest it is present within 0.5–3.8 % of benign breast biopsies [51].

The management of these lesions when diagnosed by core needle biopsy (CNB) is currently in evolution. Historically, the rates of upstage to DCIS or invasive cancer at time of excisional biopsy in these patients ranged 0–60 %, resulting in routine surgical excision after CNB for both ALH and LCIS. Inherent selection bias and lack of radiographic–pathologic correlation in many of these retrospective analyses complicate the decision regarding need for excision. Newer retrospective series suggest upgrade rates are less than 5 %, which may allow for selected patients to be spared surgical excision [52, 53]. A recent prospective multi-institutional study evaluated 74 patients with lobular neoplasia; all lesions were concordant on imaging and excision. On central pathology review, only one patient was upgraded to malignancy (1 %). This is comparable to the expected risk of breast cancer with a BI-RADS 3 mammogram reading (<2 %). The authors concluded that routine excision is not warranted, and imaging may be appropriate for some patients with lobular neoplasia [54].

The decision whether to excise these lesions should be made after careful review using a multimodality approach, with assessment of radiographic–pathologic correlation. In patients who do not undergo excisional biopsy, it is crucial to perform close surveillance, with short-term follow-up mammography.

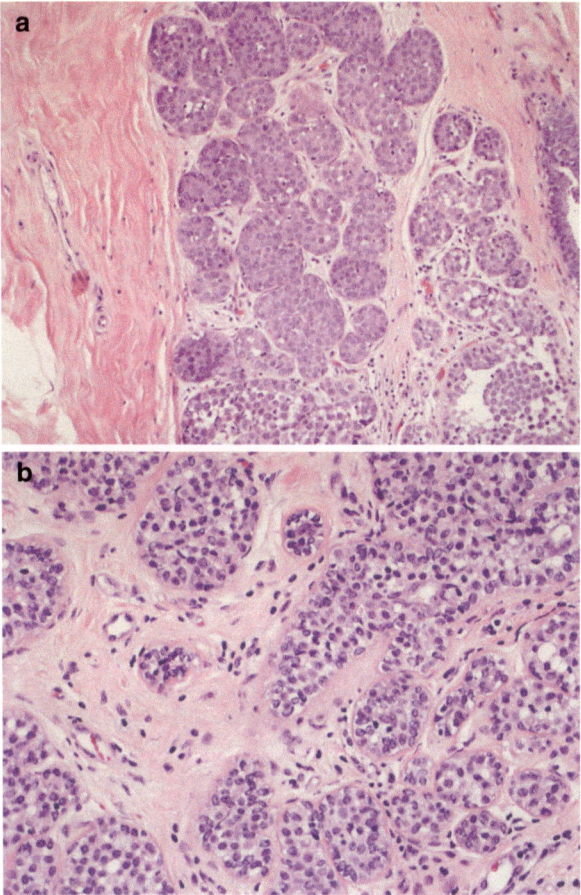

Fig. 6.5 (**a**) Lobular carcinoma in situ (magnification 200×). (**b**) Lobular carcinoma in situ (magnification 400×). The lobule is entirely replaced and mildly expanded by neoplastic cells. Individual expanded acini are distinctly visible. Some discohesion is apparent (special recognition to Paul Musto M.D., Department of Pathology, for providing pathology slides and explanations)

6.6.1   Future Cancer Risk

Patients with lobular neoplasia are at increased risk of developing breast cancer, and the magnitude of risk differs between ALH and LCIS. A recent meta-analysis of six studies reported the odds ratio (OR) of developing breast cancer as 3.92 with ALH. This is in comparison to historical data estimating an OR of 9.0 with LCIS [6, 55]. Patients with LCIS are quoted a risk of developing breast cancer at 1 % per year; this is based on data reported in 1996 by Bodian and colleagues, demonstrating 35 % risk at 35 years [56]. This risk has been confirmed with contemporary studies.

Lobular neoplasia tends to be multifocal and bilateral, and the risk of subsequent breast cancer exists in both breasts. This and the presence of both ductal and lobular phenotypes have led to assumption that ALH and LCIS were markers of increased risk. However, current data shows that the risk of subsequent breast cancer is higher in the ipsilateral breast (2:1 ratio), and these lesions share clonal proliferations similar to adjacent cancers. This has revived the debate of marker of increased risk vs. non-obligate precursor [49].

6.7   Long-Term Management of Proliferative Lesions with Atypia

6.7.1   Surveillance

At the very least, patients with proliferative breast disease exhibiting increased breast cancer risk should undergo annual mammography with clinical breast exam every 6–12 months as recommended by the National Comprehensive Cancer Network (NCCN) guidelines [57].

Contrast-enhanced breast magnetic resonance imaging (MRI) has been shown to be a valuable addition to the screening regimen for genetic mutation carriers and women at highest risk. This has prompted a recommendation of annual screening MRI in women with estimated lifetime risk greater than 20 %, as estimated by models focusing on family history [58]. Depending on the age at presentation, women with some of these proliferative lesions (especially LCIS) may have an estimated lifetime risk of breast cancer greater than 20 %. This has led to the question whether screening MRI would be of clinical benefit in these patients.

There are no randomized trials addressing this question; data consists of single institution retrospective series. Port et al. first evaluated the use of screening MRI in women with high-risk pathology. In the cohort of women with atypical hyperplasia, the group screened with MRI underwent significantly more biopsies, and no occult cancers were detected [59]. Schwartz and colleagues confirmed these findings. In 131 patients with atypical hyperplasia screened with MRI, 23.7 % of patients underwent second-look imaging and possible biopsy, and cancer was found in only two patients (1.5 %). The positive predictive value of MRI in that series of 131 patients was only 20 % [60]. Both series concluded that the low positive predictive value of MRI did not provide any added benefit over annual mammography women with atypical hyperplasia.

King and colleagues at Memorial Sloan Kettering Cancer Center reported the largest retrospective series of screening MRI in women with LCIS. In their cohort, 455 women with LCIS underwent screening MRI, compared to 321 followed with standard imaging. Women screened with MRI were more likely to be younger, premenopausal, and have at least one first-degree relative with breast cancer ($p < 0.001$). At median follow-up of 58 months, the incidence of cancer was 13 % in both groups; there was no increase in cancer detection in the group screened with MRI. Women screened with MRI were more likely to undergo at least one benign breast biopsy during the surveillance period (36 % with MRI compared to 13 %

Table 6.4 Benefit of chemoprevention in patients with atypical hyperplasia (AH) and lobular carcinoma in situ (LCIS)

Study	Experimental group	Follow-up (years)	Reduction in breast cancer incidence with chemoprevention
NSABP P-1 Fisher, 2005 [62]	Tamoxifen	7	AH RR 0.25 (95 % CI, 0.1–0.52) LCIS RR 0.54 (95 % CI, 0.27–1.02)
MAP.3 Goss, 2011 [64]	Exemestane	2.9	AH and LCIS HR 0.61 (95 % CI, 0.20–1.8)
IBIS-II Cuzick, 2014 [65]	Anastrozole	5	AH and LCIS HR 0.31 (95 % CI, 0.12–0.84)

standard imaging, $p<0.0001$). Furthermore, only 50 % of the biopsies within the MRI group were prompted by MRI findings alone. Although a trend to smaller tumor size was seen in women screened with MRI (0.5 cm in MRI group vs. 0.95 cm in standard group, $p=0.09$), there was no difference in stage or histology between the groups. The authors concluded that the decision to use breast MRI as a screening adjunct should not be based on history of LCIS alone [61].

6.7.2 Risk Reduction

The beneficial effect of chemoprevention in patients with atypical hyperplasia and LCIS has been well established by large prospective randomized trials (Table 6.4). The National Surgical Adjuvant Breast and Bowel Project (NSABP) P-1 prevention trial compared 5 years of tamoxifen to placebo in high-risk women. A significant reduction in cumulative rate of DCIS and invasive breast cancers was demonstrated with the use of tamoxifen in all subgroups of patients within the cohort. Women with atypical hyperplasia were found to have the most benefit, with 75 % reduction in invasive breast cancers at 7-year follow-up (95 % CI 0.10–0.52) [62]. The NSABP performed a second prevention trial comparing raloxifene with tamoxifen in a similar high-risk population; raloxifene was found to be slightly inferior to tamoxifen, but still reduced invasive breast cancers by approximately 38 % in postmenopausal women [63].

Furthermore, aromatase inhibitors as chemopreventive agents have also been studied in prospective randomized controlled trials. The MAP.3 trial demonstrated a 39 % reduction in breast cancers with 5 years of exemestane in postmenopausal women with history of atypical hyperplasia and LCIS [64]. In the IBIS-II trial, the use of anastrozole was also associated with significant benefit, reducing incidence of breast cancers by 53 %, with largest benefit in women with atypical hyperplasia [65]. Although both studies show promising results, median follow-up was less than 5 years, so additional data is warranted to confirm the benefit of aromatase inhibitors.

The findings of these chemoprevention trials were validated in an observational study of 2459 women with high-risk lesions, including atypical hyperplasia and LCIS. This was the first evaluation outside the context of a randomized clinical trial. The authors concluded that the use of chemoprevention was associated with a

Table 6.5 Risk reduction with the use of chemoprevention (CP) in patients with atypical lesions of the breast as reported by an observational study with 10-year follow-up [66]

	No.	5-year risk	10-year risk	
All	2459	8.3 % without CP 4.1 % with CP	21.3 % without CP 7.5 % with CP	$p<0.0001$
ADH	1198	4.8 % without CP 1.4 % with CP	19.9 % without CP 8.5 % with CP	$p<0.05$
ALH	827	11.4 % without CP 5.6 % with CP	18.7 % without CP 8.5 % with CP	$p<0.05$
LCIS	568	12.4 % without CP 7.9 % with CP	32.4 % without CP 10.2 % with CP	$p<0.05$

clinical benefit in all subgroups, reducing the incidence of breast cancer by 50 % at 5 years and 65 % at 10 years ($p<0.001$, Table 6.5) [66].

Although the benefit of chemoprevention is widely established, there is significant variation in acceptance rates as reported by institutional series. A meta-analysis reported an overall acceptance rate of 14.8 %, although this can vary from 4 to 54 %. It appears that patients who are counseled in a high-risk clinic setting may be more likely to begin therapy. Patients with LCIS are seven times more likely to initiate chemoprevention than other high-risk patients [66, 67]. It is estimated that approximately 60 % of patients who begin chemoprevention will complete the recommended 5 years of therapy. Adverse effects of hot flashes and vaginal bleeding are most common reasons for cessation of therapy [67].

Retrospective cohort studies have indicated that bilateral prophylactic mastectomy (BPM) reduces cancer development by 90 % in high-risk women based on family history [68]. Women with LCIS are at the highest risk of developing breast cancer, and BPM may be an appropriate option for a subset of women with LCIS, especially in the presence of family history or other risk factors. While BPM is effective in reducing cancer risk, it is important to counsel patients that it is irreversible and associated with risks, including surgical complications and psychosocial impact [69]. While most patients do not choose this option, results from a retrospective analysis of the Surveillance, Epidemiology, and End Results database suggest the number of women undergoing BPM for LCIS is increasing. In 14,048 women with LCIS in the cohort, the proportion of patients undergoing mastectomy increased from 12 to 15 % from 2000 to 2009 ($p<0.01$) [70].

For women who are not interested in pursuing the above strategies, there are lifestyle modifications that may be of benefit. Postmenopausal women taking hormone replacement therapy may consider cessation of these medications, as data from the Women's Health Initiative Study showed a 26 % increase in incidence of breast cancer in women taking combined hormone therapy [71]. This study did not see an increase in incidence with estrogen alone, although other studies have shown the use of estrogen only as hormone replacement is associated with increased risk [72, 73].

Numerous studies have shown that even light to moderate alcohol intake can be associated with an increase in breast cancer risk, prompting the NCCN Breast Cancer Risk Reduction Panel to recommend alcohol consumption be limited to <1 drink per day [57]. Maintenance of a healthy body mass index may reduce risk, as there is also data indicating that overweight and obese women are at an increased risk. Data from the Nurses' Health Study showed that weight gain greater than 25 kg after age 18 was associated with 45 % increase in breast cancer risk [74]. Regular exercise can reduce this risk, as multiple population-based studies showed a reduction in breast cancer risk in women who participate in vigorous exercise on a weekly basis [57].

6.8 Conclusion

Proliferative lesions are associated with an increased risk of breast cancer development as shown by epidemiological studies. These lesions are relatively common findings on core biopsies for either mammographic abnormalities or palpable findings. Not all of these lesions diagnosed by core biopsy mandate surgical excision. The data suggests some of these lesions have low probability of upstage to cancer, and there may be some patients who are appropriate candidates for short-term follow-up imaging in lieu of surgical excision. Decisions regarding need for surgical excision should be made after careful review of imaging findings and pathology results to determine concordance. Once the diagnosis has been established, counseling regarding future risk of breast cancer should be performed. In this population of patients, there does not appear to be data confirming benefit of screening MRI over standard imaging modalities. One can consider risk reduction strategies such as lifestyle modifications, chemoprevention, and bilateral prophylactic mastectomy in appropriate patients.

References

1. Worsham MJ, Abrams J, Raju U, Kapke A, Liu M, Cheng P, et al. Breast cancer incidence in a cohort of women with benign breast disease from a multiethnic, primary care population. Breast J. 2007;13(2):115–21.
2. National Comprehensive Cancer Network. Breast Cancer Screening and Diagnosis (Version 1.2015). http://www.nccn.org/professionals/physician_gls/pdf/breast-screening.pdf. Accessed 17 July 2015.
3. Dupont W, Page D. Risk factors for breast cancer in women with proliferative breast disease. NEJM. 1985;312(3):146–51.
4. Collins L, Baer H, Tamimi R, Connolly J, Colditz G, Schnitt S. Magnitude and laterality of breast cancer risk according to histologic type of atypical hyperplasia: results from the nurses' health study. Cancer. 2007;109(2):180–7.
5. Zhou W, Xue D, Liu X, Ding Q, Wang S. The influence of family history and biological stratification on breast cancer risk in women with benign breast disease: a meta-analysis. J Cancer Res Clin Oncol. 2011;137:1053–60.
6. Dyrstad S, Yan Y, Fowler A, Colditz G. Breast cancer risk associated with benign breast disease: systematic review and meta-analysis. Breast Cancer Res Treat. 2015;149:569–75.
7. Georgian-Smith D, Lawton T. Controversies on the management of high risk lesions at core biopsy from a radiology/pathology perspective. Radiol Clin N Am. 2010;48:999–1012.

8. Said S, Visscher D, Nassar A, Frank R, Vierkant R, Frost M, et al. Flat epithelial atypia and risk of breast cancer: a mayo cohort study. Cancer. 2015;121:1548–55.

9. Uzoaru I, Morgan B, Liu Z, Bellafiore F, Gaudier F, Lo J, et al. Flat epithelial atypia with and without atypical ductal hyperplasia: to excise or not. Results of a 5-year prospective study. Virchows Arch. 2012;461:419–23.

10. Calhoun B, Sobel A, White R, Gromet M, Flippo T, Sarantou T, et al. Management of flat epithelial atypia on breast core biopsy may be individualized based on correlation with imaging studies. Mod Pathol. 2015;28:670–6.

11. Desouki M, Li Z, Fadare O, Zhou C. Incidental atypical proliferative lesions in reduction mammoplasty specimens: analysis from 2498 cases from 2 tertiary women's health centers. Hum Pathol. 2013;44(9):1877–81.

12. Verschuur-Maes A, van Deurzen C, Monninkhof E, van Diest P. Columnar cell lesions on breast needle biopsies: is surgical excision necessary? A systematic review. Ann Surg. 2012;255(2):259–65.

13. Moinfar F, Man Y, Bratthauer G, Ratschek M, Tavassoli F. Genetic abnormalities in mammary ductal intraepithelial neoplasia-flat type ("Clinging Ductal Carcinoma In Situ"). Cancer. 2000;88(9):2072–81.

14. Tabar L, Dean PB. Stellate lesions. In: Teaching atlas of mammography. 2nd ed. New York: Georg Theime Verlag; 1985. p. 87–136.

15. Krishnamurthy S, Bevers T, Kuerer H, Yang W. Multidisciplinary considerations in the management of high risk breast lesions. AJR. 2012;198(2):132–40.

16. Kennedy M, Masterson A, Kerin M, Flanagan F. Pathology and clinical relevance of radial scars: a review. J Clin Pathol. 2003;56:721–4.

17. Conlon N, D'Arcy C, Kaplan J, Bowser Z, Cordero A, Brogi E, et al. Radial scar at image-guided needle biopsy: is excision necessary? Am J Surg Pathol. 2015;39(6):779–85.

18. Sloane J, Mayers N. Carcinoma and atypical hyperplasia in radial scars and complex sclerosing lesions: importance of lesion size and patient age. Histopathology. 1993;23:225–31.

19. Manfrin E, Remo A, Falsirollo F, Reghellin D, Bonetti F. Risk of neoplastic transformation in asymptomatic radial scar: analysis of 117 cases. Breast Cancer Res Treat. 2008;107:371–7.

20. Matrai C, D'Alfonso T, Pharmer L, Drotman M, Simmons R, Shin S. Advocating non-surgical management of patients with small, incidental radial scars at time of needle core biopsy. Arch Pathol Lab Med. 2015;139(9):1137–42 (epub).

21. Nassar A, Conners A, Celik B, Jenkins S, Smith C, Hieken T. Radial scar/complex sclerosing lesions: a clinicopathologic correlation study from a single institution. Ann Diagn Pathol. 2015;19(1):24–8.

22. Resetkova E, Edelweiss M, Albarracin C, et al. Management of radial sclerosing lesions of the breast using percutaneous vacuum-assisted core needle biopsy: recommendations for excision based on seven years' of experience at a single institution. Breast Cancer Res Treat. 2011;127:335–43.

23. Brenner R, Jackman R, Parker S, Evans W, Philpotts L, Deutch B, et al. Percutaneous core needle biopsy of radial scars of the breast: when is excision necessary? AJR. 2002; 179:1179–84.

24. Jacobs T, Byrne C, Colditz G, Connoly J, Schnitt S. Radial scars in benign breast biopsy specimens and the risk of breast cancer. NEJM. 1999;340(6):430–6.

25. Sanders M, Page D, Simpson J, Schuyler P, Plummer W, Dupont W. Interdependence of radial scar and proliferative disease with respect to invasive carcinoma risk in patients with benign breast biopsies. Cancer. 2006;106(7):1453–61.

26. Berg J, Visscher D, Vierkant R, Pankratz V, Maloney S, Lewis J, et al. Breast cancer risk in women with radial scars in benign breast biopsies. Breast Cancer Res Treat. 2008;108(2):167–74.

27. Amin A, Purdy A, Mattingly J, Kong A. Benign breast disease. Surg Clin N Am. 2013; 93:299–308.

28. Rizzo M, Linebarger J, Lowe M, Pan L, Gabram S, Vasquez L, et al. Management of papillary breast lesions diagnosed on core needle biopsy: clinical pathologic and radiologic analysis of 276 cases with surgical follow up. J Am Chem Soc. 2012;214(3):280–7.

29. Lewis J, Hartmann L, Vierkant R, Maloney S, Pankratz S, Allers T, et al. An analysis of breast cancer risk in women with single, multiple, and atypical papilloma. Am J Surg Pathol. 2006;30(6):665–72.
30. Eiada R, Chong J, Kulkarni S, Goldberg F, Muradali F. Papillary lesions of the breast: MRI, ultrasound, and mammographic appearances. AJR. 2012;198(2):264–71.
31. Wen X, Cheng W. Non-malignant breast papillary lesions at core needle biopsy: a meta-analysis of underestimation and influencing factors. Ann Surg Oncol. 2013;20:94–101.
32. McGhan L, Pockaj B, Wasif N, Giurescu M, McCullough A, Gray R. Papillary lesions on core breast biopsy: excisional biopsy for all patients? Am Surg. 2013;79(12):1238–42.
33. Jaffer S, Bleiweis I, Nagi C. Incidental intraductal papillomas (<2 mm) of the breast diagnosed on needle core biopsy do not need to be excised. Breast J. 2013;19:130–3.
34. Weisman P, Sutton B, Siziopikou K, Hansen N, Khan S, Neuschler E, et al. Non-mass-associated intraductal papillomas: is excision necessary? Hum Pathol. 2014;45:583–8.
35. Shamonki J, Chung A, Huynh K, Sim M, Kinnaird S, Guiliano A. Management of papillary lesions of the breast: can larger core needle biopsy samples identify patients who may avoid surgical excision? Ann Surg Oncol. 2013;20:4137–44.
36. Wyss P, Varga Z, Rossle M, Rageth C. Papillary lesions of the breast: outcomes of 156 patients managed without excisional biopsy. Breast J. 2014;20(4):394–401.
37. Mosier A, Keylock J, Smith D. Benign papillomas diagnosed on large-gauge vacuum-assisted core needle biopsy which span <1.5 cm do not need surgical excision. Breast J. 2013;19(6):611–7.
38. Swapp R, Glazebrook K, Jones K, Brandts H, Reynolds C, Visscher D, et al. Management of benign intraductal solitary papilloma diagnosed on core needle biopsy. Ann Surg Oncol. 2013;20:1900–5.
39. Mesurolle B, Perez J, Azzumea F, Lemercier E, Xie X, Aldis A, et al. Atypical ductal hyperplasia diagnosed at sonographically guided core needle biopsy: frequency, final surgical outcome, and factors associated with underestimation. AJR. 2014;202:1389–94.
40. Pearlman M, Griffin J. Benign breast disease. Obstet Gynecol. 2010;116:747–58.
41. Polom K, Murawa D, Kurzawa P, Michalak M, Murawa P. Underestimation of cancer in case of diagnosis of atypical ductal hyperplasia (ADH) by vacuum assisted core needle biopsy. Rep Pract Oncol Radiother. 2012;17:129–33.
42. Dominici L, Liao G, Brock J, Iglehart J, Lotfi P, Meyer J, et al. Large needle core biopsy of atypical ductal hyperplasia: results of surgical excision. Breast J. 2012;18(5):506–8.
43. Nguyen C, Albarracin C, Whitman G, Lopez A, Sneige N. Atypical ductal hyperplasia in directional vacuum-assisted biopsy of breast microcalcifications: considerations for surgical excision. Ann Surg Oncol. 2011;18(3):752–61.
44. Villa A, Tagliafico A, Chiesa F, Chiaramondia M, Friedman D, Calabrese M. Atypical ductal hyperplasia diagnosed at 11-guage vacuum-assisted breast biopsy performed on suspicious clustered microcalcifications: could patients without residual microcalcifications be managed conservatively? AJR. 2011;197:1012–8.
45. Heller S, Moy L. Imaging features and management of high-risk lesions on contrast-enhanced dynamic breast MRI. AJR. 2012;198:245–55.
46. Linda A, Zuiani C, Furlan A, Lorenzon M, Londero V, Girometti R, et al. Nonsurgical management of high-risk lesions diagnosed at core needle biopsy: can malignancy be ruled out safely with breast MRI? AJR. 2012;198:272–80.
47. Degnim A, Visscher D, Berman H, Frost M, Sellers T, Vierkant R, et al. Stratification of breast cancer risk in women with atypia: a Mayo Cohort Study. JCO. 2007;25(19):2671–7.
48. Hartmann L, Radisky D, Frost M, Santen R, Vierkant R, Benetti L, et al. Understanding the premalignant potential of atypical hyperplasia through its natural history: a Longitudinal Cohort Study. Cancer Prev Res. 2014;7(2):211–7.
49. King T, Reis-Filho J. Lobular carcinoma in situ: biology and management. In: Harris J, Lippman M, Morrow M, Osborne C, editors. Diseases of the breast. Philadelphia: Wolters Kluwer Health; 2014. p. 324–36.
50. Jorns J, Sabel M, Pang J. Lobular neoplasia: morphology and management. Arch Pathol Lab Med. 2014;138:1344–9.

51. Oppong B, King T. Recommendations for women with Lobular Carcinoma In Situ (LCIS). Oncology (Williston Park). 2011;25(11):1051–6.
52. Rendi M, Dintzis S, Lehman C, Calhoun K, Allison K. Lobular in-situ neoplasia on breast core needle biopsy: imaging indications and pathologic extent can identify which patients require excisional biopsy. Ann Surg Oncol. 2012;19:914–21.
53. Murray M, Luedtke C, Liberman L, Nehhozina T, Akram M, Brogi E. Classic lobular carcinoma in situ and atypical lobular hyperplasia at percutaneous breast core biopsy: outcomes of prospective excision. Cancer. 2013;119:1073–9.
54. Nakhlis F, Gilmore L, Gelman R, King T, Bedrosian I, Ludwig K, et al. The incidence of adjacent synchronous invasive carcinoma and/or DCIS in patients with lobular neoplasia on core biopsy: results from a prospective multi-institutional registry (TBCRC 020). Submitted. Ann Surg Oncol. 2016 Mar;23(3):722–8. doi:10.1245/s10434-015-4922-4. Epub 2015 Nov 5.
55. Page D, Kidd T, Dupont W, Simpson J, Rogers L. Lobular neoplasia of the breast: higher risk for subsequent invasive cancer predicted by more extensive disease. Hum Pathol. 1991; 22:1232–9.
56. Bodian C, Perzin K, Lattes R. Lobular neoplasia. Cancer. 1996;78:1024–34.
57. National Comprehensive Cancer Network. Breast Cancer Risk Reduction (Version 2.2015). http://www.nccn.org/professionals/physician_gls/pdf/breast_risk.pdf. Accessed 12 July 2015.
58. Saslow D, Boetes C, Burke W, Harms S, Leach M, Lehmann C, et al. American cancer society guidelines for breast screening with MRI as an adjunct to mammography. CA Cancer J Clin. 2007;57:75–89.
59. Port E, Park A, Borgen P, Morris E, Montgomery L. Results of MRI screening for breast cancer in high-risk patients with LCIS and atypical hyperplasia. Ann Surg Oncol. 2007; 14(3):1051–7.
60. Schwartz T, Cyr A, Margenthaler J. Screening breast magnetic resonance imaging in women with atypia or lobular carcinoma in situ. J Surg Res. 2015;193:519–22.
61. King T, Muhsen S, Patil S, Koskow S, Oskar S, Park A, et al. Is there a role for screening MRI in women with LCIS? Breast Cancer Res Treat. 2013;142(2):445–53.
62. Fisher B, Costantino J, Wickerham D, Cecchini R, Cronin W, Robidoux A, et al. Tamoxifen for the prevention of breast cancer: current status of the national surgical adjuvant breast and bowel project P-1 study. JNCI. 2005;97(22):1652–62.
63. Vogel V, Costantino J, Wickerham D, Cronin W, Cecchini R, Atkins J, et al. Update of national surgical adjuvant breast and bowel project Study of Tamoxifen and Raloxifene (STAR) P-2 trial: preventing breast cancer. Cancer Prev Res. 2010;3(6):696–706.
64. Goss P, Ingle J, Ales-Martinez J, Cheung A, Chlebowski R, Wactawski-Wende J, et al. Exemestane for breast-cancer prevention in postmenopausal women. NEJM. 2011;364: 2381–91.
65. Cuzick J, Sestak I, Forbes J, Dowsett M, Knox J, Cawthorn S, et al. Anastrozole for prevention of breast cancer in high-risk postmenopausal women (IBIS-II): an international, double-blind, randomized placebo-controlled trial. Lancet. 2014;383:1041–2.
66. Coopey S, Mazzola E, Buckley J, Sharko J, Belli A, Kim E, et al. The role of chemoprevention in modifying the risk of breast cancer in women with atypical breast lesions. Breast Cancer Res Treat. 2012;136:627–33.
67. Roetzheim R, Lee J, Fulp W, Gomez E, Clayton E, Tollin S, et al. Acceptance and adherence to chemoprevention among women at increased risk of breast cancer. Breast. 2015; 24:51–6.
68. Hartmann L, Schaid D, Woods J, Crotty T, Myers J, Arnold P, et al. Efficacy of bilateral prophylactic mastectomy in women with a family history of breast cancer. NEJM. 1999;340(2):77–84.
69. Burke E, Portschy P, Tuttle T. Prophylactic mastectomy: who needs it, when and why. J Surg Oncol. 2015;111:91–5.

70. Portschy P, Marmor S, Nzara R, Virnig B, Tuttle T. Trends in incidence and management of lobular carcinoma in situ: a population-based analysis. Ann Surg Oncol. 2013;20: 3240–6.
71. Rossouw J, Anderson G, Prentice R, LaCroix A, Kooperber C, Stefanick M, et al. Risks and benefits of estrogen plus progestin in healthy postmenopausal women. JAMA. 2002;288(3): 321–33.
72. Beral V. Breast cancer and hormone-replacement therapy in the Million Women Study. Lancet. 2003;362:419–27.
73. Chen W, Manson J, Hankinson S, Rosner B, Holmes W, Willett W, et al. Unopposed estrogen therapy and the risk of invasive breast cancer. Arch Intern Med. 2006;166:1027–32.
74. Eliassen A, Colditz G, Rosner B, Willett W, Hankinson S. Adult weight change and risk of postmenopausal breast cancer. JAMA. 2006;296(2):193–201.

Chapter 7
Approach to Imaging

Hal Douglas Kipfer

7.1 Introduction

Screening women at high risk for breast cancer continues to evolve as new evidence is published. More uncertainty has been introduced recently by enactment of breast density notification laws in 23 states [1]. The purpose of this chapter is to give front-line providers a basis for discussing high-risk screening options with their patients. It is important to note that the USPSTF guidelines [2] (with update in progress) do not address the high-risk screening population. The 2007 American Cancer Society Guidelines serve as the foundation for high-risk screening [3]. This chapter also reports new data that have been published since those guidelines with regard to additional high-risk patients. Finally, since the literature continues to grow more quickly that texts can be published, concepts useful in evaluation of screening tests will be covered with discussion of risks, benefits, and limitations of each imaging modality. Issues of cost, radiation dose, breast density, and other factors will be summarized for each type of imaging.

7.2 Patient Risk Input

Some assumptions will be made about the risk assessment that precedes this chapter, and some organizing principles are worth reviewing. Screening high-risk women, defined as greater than 20 % estimated lifetime risk, is relatively simple: annual mammography plus MRI, with ultrasound reserved for women who have contraindications to MRI. The more difficult task is trying to ascertain who else may benefit from the addition of MRI when the risk prediction models do not reach 20 %.

H.D. Kipfer, MD
Department of Radiology, Indiana Radiology Partners, Indianapolis, IN, USA
e-mail: refpikh@gmail.com

© Springer International Publishing Switzerland 2016
L.A. Mina et al. (eds.), *Breast Cancer Prevention and Treatment*,
DOI 10.1007/978-3-319-19437-0_7

7.2.1   Lifetime Risk

Since lifetime risk is a cumulative measure, it is important to understand that it decreases for any given patient as she ages. Many of the risk numbers that we consider for making screening decisions are quoted as percent estimated lifetime risk.

7.2.2   5- and 10-Year Risk

While lifetime risk decreases with age, the likelihood that a given woman will get breast cancer in an upcoming interval, such as 5- and 10-year risk, increases with age [4]. At first glance, this may seem counterintuitive. Another way to help make sense of the relationship between lifetime risk and 10-year risk is to consider lifetime risk as the sum of all the 10-year risks that a patient will have during her life. So any given decade's risk will be lower than lifetime risk, but the 10-year risk increases with each successive decade. There does seem to be a plateau in age-specific incidence around the seventh decade, but mortality continues to increase [5].

7.3   Modality Overview

7.3.1   Mammography

Full-field digital mammography (FFDM) is a specialized, widely available, radiographic evaluation of the breasts. As of mid-2015, the FDA reports 14,136 of the total 14,600 (96.8 %) mammography units in the United States are digital. Mammography is still the only screening modality with proven mortality reduction, with randomized controlled trial (RTC) meta-analyses showing a 20 % decrease in mortality. RTC metadata are also likely to underestimate screening for multiple reasons. One reason is selection bias in the Canadian trials that resulted in women with palpable abnormalities disproportionately being assigned to the screening group. Another is cross-contamination of uninvited women getting screened outside the trial and invited women failing to participate. Regardless of how the data are parsed, mammography is considered the standard for breast cancer screening in high-risk women. While the starting age and frequency of screening are hotly debated in average-risk women, high-risk women should have screening mammography performed annually, usually beginning before age 40, but rarely beginning before age 25 [6].

As a general principle, it makes sense to start mammography in high-risk women when their 5-year risk equals that of an average 40-year-old. However, it is difficult to apply this in daily practice. A more practical practice says that women with greater than 20 % estimated lifetime risk should start between ages 25 and 30 years. Women with a diagnosis of atypia or LCIS on a biopsy before age 40 should continue annual screening mammography thereafter. The same holds true for women with a personal history of breast cancer treated by breast conservation therapy.

7.3.2   Tomosynthesis

Digital breast tomosynthesis (DBT), often referred to as 3D mammography, was first approved by the FDA in 2009 and first reimbursed by Centers for Medicare and Medicaid Services (CMS) in 2015. DBT utilizes multiple low-dose images taken at varying angles over the breast, which are then reconstructed into thin slices to reduce the effect of overlying tissues that can obscure cancers. This has resulted in the ability to detect more invasive cancers and reduce the number of false positives at screening [7]. Cancer detection increases as high as 53 % have been shown and reductions in recall rates have been similar [8]. Fewer women recalled with more cancers detected are a win-win outcome that is often difficult to achieve in medicine. 3D mammography is usually done in conjunction with standard 2D full-field digital mammography (FFDM); however, the 2D views can be synthesized from the 3D data set, which allows for decreased radiation exposure.

Aside from the increased capital costs of DBT equipment, interpretation times are also increased. These factors combined with limited reimbursement have also resulted in limited availability, but there are suggestions that technology adoption will continue to increase [9, 10]. Radiation dose is also increased when 2D and 3D are done in combination, but synthesized 2D views should help offset this with time [8].

Ultimately, the added benefit of DBT in high-risk women is uncertain, if they are getting their recommended screening MRI. Further, BRCA mutation carriers may want to limit radiation exposure as they may be more sensitive to ionizing radiation-related changes to DNA [11].

7.3.3   MRI

7.3.3.1 2007 American Cancer Society (ACS) Guidelines

The 2007 ACS guidelines for MRI screening of breast cancer have been widely published [3]. *Should they be reproduced here or in risk assessment chapters?*

7.3.3.2 New Since Guidelines

2007 ACS guidelines stated that there was insufficient evidence to add screening breast MRI in women with a personal history of breast cancer. Since then, a small retrospective study found a cancer detection rate of 18.1 additional cancers per 1000 women screened [12]. While this detection rate is comparable to published high-risk screening results [13], the study is admittedly small. Still, MRI screening of women with a personal history of breast cancer, who are treated with breast conserving therapy, warrants consideration and further study.

Personal history of atypia on percutaneous biopsy was also placed in the insufficient evidence group in the 2007 ACS guidelines. However, large cohort studies suggest estimated lifetime risk of >30 % in women with history of atypia [14]. Since this is well above the 20 % threshold in the guidelines, these women should strongly consider the addition of screening breast MRI to their surveillance plans.

MRI is not affected by breast density or volume of fibroglandular tissue, so as risk increases, breast MRI becomes more effective and has the highest supplemental yield of any of the current test options. The more difficult question is whether increased breast density alone is sufficient reason to add breast MRI. Further complicating this question is the information mandated by breast density notification that is currently binary—dense or not dense. This means that a woman with 49 % breast density would not be involved in the density and risk discussion, whereas a woman with 51 % density would receive the same information as a woman with 99 % density.

7.3.3.3 Future Applications of Breast MRI

Abbreviated breast MRI techniques are being evaluated and show promise for reducing the time and expense involved in using MRI as a screening tool, without significant decreases in accuracy [15]. Further study is required, but as MRI gets more cost-effective, more women should be able to benefit from MR's superior performance. This could result in a shift in the estimated lifetime risk threshold to 15 %, for example. Improvements in imaging techniques will hopefully accelerate and facilitate these changes [16, 17].

Background parenchymal enhancement (BPE) is the extent that the overall breast tissue enhances, or lights up, after administration of gadolinium-based contrast materials. BPE is being investigated as an independent risk factor for developing breast cancer, and notably, BPE decreases in women taking aromatase inhibitors and SERMs [18–20]. BPE may be a more accurate predictor of risk than mammographic breast density [21]. Much like breast density though, we lack consistent methods to quantify BPE, and it is not incorporated into current risk prediction models.

Breast MRI may be an ideal method to lessen the burden of overdiagnosis and overtreatment on patients with breast cancer. Much more study is needed, but in the future, we hope to spare some patients from needing to receive cytotoxic, surgical, and radiation therapies by more accurately identifying those who respond to treatment and prophylactic therapies. This is beyond the scope of the high-risk screening discussion, but it highlights other potential ways that MRI might someday benefit high-risk women.

Estimation of glandular volume would likely be much more accurate on breast MRI than mammography because of the high tissue contrast and cross-sectional nature of MRI. However, given the apparent greater importance of BPE, this may not yield much benefit in patient risk stratification for screening and prophylactic decision-making. Still, it may improve our ability to quantify mammographic breast density if we can better understand and correlate MRI and mammographic glandular volumes.

7.3.4 Ultrasound

Screening breast ultrasound data continue to accrue, making any static assessment difficult. However, in simplest terms, one thing is clear early on: women with risk profiles similar to the ACRIN 6666 population should not have screening breast ultrasound unless they have a contraindication to screening breast MRI, since the supplemental yield of MRI was 14.7 per 1000 after normal mammography plus ultrasound [22]. The more difficult question is whether increased breast density adds enough additional risk to meet the screening MRI threshold. The Connecticut experience suggests that screening women with dense breasts with ultrasound yielded a cancer detection rate of 1.8 cancers per 1000 women with normal mammograms [23]. An automated whole-breast ultrasound (AWBUS) screening study found 1.9 cancers per 1000 in addition to the 5.4 cancers per 1000 found by mammography, suggesting that mammography finds 74 % of cancers in the setting of dense breast for average-risk women. However, the cost per cancer detected by ultrasound was essentially tripled, largely due to the low positive predictive values (PPV) and excess biopsies [24].

Whole-breast screening in the ACRIN 6666 trial was performed by breast radiologists (physicians) with handheld ultrasound transducers. The advantage is that this ultrasound equipment is widely available in existing breast imaging practices. However, this practice is very resource intensive with physicians scanning the patients. Automated breast (AB) ultrasound (US) is increasingly available and as noted above is associated with increased costs and false positives. Again, handheld or AB ultrasound should not be recommended in high-risk women, unless they cannot have MRI.

7.3.5 Nuclear Imaging

Positron emission mammography (PEM) and breast-specific gamma imaging (BSGI) have been studied as breast screening modalities with promising results in terms of sensitivity and specificity. However, the radiation doses to the organs that clear these radiotracers from the body are currently considered (by many) to be too high for routine use in screening. Given the lack of widespread availability of PEM and BSGI and the lack of superiority to breast MRI [25], the use at this time is probably best restricted to research applications. Leading researchers do continue to improve the technique, and if whole-body dose and availability issues can be overcome, these may be viable tools in the future.

7.4 Radiation Dose

Some dose considerations are mentioned elsewhere, but they are summarized here.

MRI and ultrasound do not use ionizing radiation, so dose is not relevant to these two.

Mammography and tomosynthesis do use ionizing radiation. However, radiation dose for digital mammography is lower than older, now virtually obsolete film-screen techniques. While tomosynthesis roughly doubled dose in its first iteration, newer software is allowing DBT to be done at doses roughly equal to 2D mammography. It is also important to remember that radiation dose from a mammogram is only a fraction of the natural annual background radiation that we all receive just living on earth. It is also interesting that we do not see significantly increased risk of breast cancer in women treated with mantle radiation after the age of 40. Finally, it is good to know that the original mammographic screening trials were done at even higher doses because they predated marked improvements in imaging equipment. The last two observations suggest that benefits of mammography are far greater than the theoretical risks of increased radiation exposure.

There may be increased risk from radiation dose in young BRCA mutation carriers. While the clinical significance of this is hard to know with certainty, it bears keeping in mind.

Dose considerations for nuclear breast imaging modalities like PEM and BSGI do not involve the breast, as much as the organ systems involved in clearing the radiotracers that are injected into the bloodstream. Specifically, the GI and urinary tracts doses, as well as whole-body doses, are currently considered by many to be too high for use as screening tool.

7.5 Invasiveness and Needle Required?

One other consideration, especially for patients who hate the thought or sight of needles, is how invasive a test can be. Mammography and ultrasound themselves do not require needles. MRI requires an IV line for administration of gadolinium contrast. Invasiveness of a biopsy is essentially the same regardless of imaging guidance needed to locate the abnormality. However, ultrasound results in a marked increase in the number of biopsies that need to be performed—as high as 20 biopsies to find one cancer. DBT has a slight edge over FFDM and MRI, but these three are all relatively close in this regard, typically finding one cancer in every 2.5 to 5 biopsies.

7.6 Density

Breast density is the newest confounder in the screening discussion. The issue is further complicated by varying state requirements for density reporting. One major shortcoming of the legislation is the arbitrary, binary separation for reporting and not-reporting density. This means that a woman with 49 % density would not be notified, but a woman with 50 % density would be. In reality, the effects of density at 49 and 50 % density are identical.

Defining density. Breast density refers to the bright tissue on a mammogram. X-rays are blocked least by fat and to a greater degree by fibrous and glandular elements within the breast. In addition, a thick band of fibroglandular tissue is brighter (blocks more X-rays) than a thin band of tissue. The most prevalent form of reporting to date is defined by the American College of Radiology (ACR) Breast Imaging and Reporting Data System (BI-RADS) [26], which is currently driven by the perceived insensitivity of mammography due to the presence of dense fibroglandular tissue. The current system splits density into four categories, A through D (previously 1 through 4), by increasing density. This method is very subjective with substantial limitations [27].

Semiquantitative, computer analysis automated techniques show promise for more consistent density assessment and are increasingly being evaluated, but are not yet widely available or standardized.

Prevalence of dense breasts. According to Breast Cancer Surveillance Consortium (BCSC) data analysis, 43.3 % (95 % confidence interval [CI] = 43.1–43.4 %) of women 40–74 years old had BI-RADS category C or D breast density [28]. These numbers are in line with our initial experience with computer-based density analysis.

Breast density issues. There are two problems with dense breasts. First, most breast cancers, like fibroglandular tissue, are bright on mammograms and can be easily obscured by dense breast tissue [29]. So mammographic sensitivity decreases as breast density increases. Sensitivities were 98 %, 82.9 %, 64.4 %, and 47.8 %, respectively, in BI-RADS density categories A, B, C, and D [30]. The second problem arising from dense breast tissue is an increased risk of developing breast cancer. Multiple studies have estimated the odds ratio of risk for developing breast cancer of 2.8–6.0, when comparing most dense breasts ($\geq$60–75 %) to least dense breasts ($\leq$0–20 %) [31]. While most people believe risk increases with density, none of the commonly used risk prediction models currently incorporate density. This means that some women who may benefit from MRI do not reach currently accepted thresholds for MRI screening, because their breast density is not included in risk calculations.

While tumor characteristics have been shown to be related to breast density [32], this does not currently affect screening decision-making.

Breast density results can also be confusing. Many women remain unaware of their breast density and the effect it has on screening [33]. However, other factors such as anxiety and insurance coverage play an equally important role in screening decisions [34, 35]. At the same time, one small study showed that primary care physicians are not all aware of density notification laws and are often not comfortable addressing questions related to breast density [36].

7.7 Putting It All Together

In the past, screening tests were looked at in a binary fashion—is cancer present or not? The new screening paradigm needs to include additional information from our screening tests into our risk assessment and risk reduction strategies. One example would be to include mammographic breast density into future risk assessments for a given patient. Maybe a woman with entirely fatty breasts finds her risk-benefit ratio favoring less expensive or less frequent screening, and a woman with extremely dense breasts and an intermediate family history may benefit from adding MRI. Effects on treatment could also help reduce side effects for patients. For example, a woman without decreased BPE on MRI after initiation of a SERM may decide that the side-effect profile she is experiencing is not worth tolerating, if we find that this lack of imaging response is a good surrogate for the risk reduction benefits of SERMs. Do not misunderstand; these are goals that require further study and not current standards of care. However, it is exciting to think that we might be able to glean additional information from our screening studies, beyond the current cancer-present-or-absent model.

7.8 Not

Guide to perform imaging
Guide to interpreting imaging

References

1. Durning MV. Breast density notification laws by state–interactive map 2015. Available from: http://www.diagnosticimaging.com/breast-imaging/breast-density-notification-laws-state-interactive-map.
2. Force USPST. Screening for breast cancer: U.S. Preventive Services Task Force recommendation statement. Ann Intern Med. 2009;151(10):716–26, W-236. doi:10.7326/0003-4819-151-10-200911170-00008.
3. Saslow D, Boetes C, Burke W, Harms S, Leach MO, Lehman CD, et al. American Cancer Society guidelines for breast screening with MRI as an adjunct to mammography. CA Cancer J Clin. 2007;57(2):75–89.
4. Graubard BI, Freedman AN, Gail MH. Five-year and lifetime risk of breast cancer among U.S. subpopulations: implications for magnetic resonance imaging screening. Cancer Epidemiol Biomark Prev Publ Am Assoc Cancer Res Cospon Am Soc Prev Oncol. 2010;19(10):2430–6. doi:10.1158/1055-9965.EPI-10-0324. PubMed PMID: 20841391, PubMed Central PMCID: PMC2952062.
5. American Cancer Society. Breast Cancer Facts & Figures 2015–2016. Atlanta: American Cancer Society, Inc. 2015.
6. Mainiero MB, Lourenco A, et al. ACR Appropriateness criteria breast cancer screening. Available at https://acsearch.acr.org/docs/70910/Narrative/. American College of Radiology. Accessed 1 May 2015.
7. Friedewald SM, Rafferty EA, Rose SL, et al. Breast cancer screening using tomosynthesis in combination with digital mammography. JAMA. 2014;311(24):2499–507. doi:10.1001/jama.2014.6095.

8. Svahn TM, Houssami N, Sechopoulos I, Mattsson S. Review of radiation dose estimates in digital breast tomosynthesis relative to those in two-view full-field digital mammography. Breast. 2014;24(2):93–9. doi:10.1016/j.breast.2014.12.002.

9. Lee CI, Lehman CD. Digital breast tomosynthesis and the challenges of implementing an emerging breast cancer screening technology into clinical practice. J Am Coll Radiol. 2013;10(12):913–7. doi:10.1016/j.jacr.2013.09.010.

10. Hardesty LA, Kreidler SM, Glueck DH. Digital breast tomosynthesis utilization in the United States: a survey of physician members of the society of breast imaging. J Am Coll Radiol. 2014;11(6):594–9. doi:10.1016/j.jacr.2013.11.025.

11. Pijpe A, Andrieu N, Easton DF, Kesminiene A, Cardis E, Nogues C, et al. Exposure to diagnostic radiation and risk of breast cancer among carriers of BRCA1/2 mutations: retrospective cohort study (GENE-RAD-RISK). BMJ. 2012;345, e5660. doi:10.1136/bmj. e5660. PubMed PMID: 22956590, PubMed Central PMCID: PMC3435441.

12. Gweon HM, Cho N, Han W, Yi A, Moon HG, Noh DY, et al. Breast MR imaging screening in women with a history of breast conservation therapy. Radiology. 2014;272(2):366–73. doi:10.1148/radiol.14131893.

13. Niell BL, Gavenonis SC, Motazedi T, Chubiz JC, Halpern EP, Rafferty EA, et al. Auditing a breast MRI practice: performance measures for screening and diagnostic breast MRI. J Am Coll Radiol. 2014;11(9):883–9. http://dx.doi.org/10.1016/j.jacr.2014.02.003.

14. Hartmann LC, Degnim AC, Santen RJ, Dupont WD, Ghosh K. Atypical hyperplasia of the breast–risk assessment and management options. N Engl J Med. 2015;372(1):78–89. doi:10.1056/NEJMsr1407164.

15. Kuhl CK, Schrading S, Strobel K, Schild HH, Hilgers RD, Bieling HB. Abbreviated breast Magnetic Resonance Imaging (MRI): first postcontrast subtracted images and maximum-intensity projection-A novel approach to breast cancer screening with MRI. J Clin Oncol Off J Am Soc Clin Oncol. 2014;32(22):2304–10. doi:10.1200/JCO.2013.52.5386.

16. Le Y, Kipfer H, Majidi S, Holz S, Dale B, Geppert C, et al. Application of time-resolved angiography with stochastic trajectories (TWIST)-Dixon in dynamic contrast-enhanced (DCE) breast MRI. J Magn Reson Imaging JMRI. 2013;38(5):1033–42. doi:10.1002/jmri.24062.

17. Mann RM, Mus RD, van Zelst J, Geppert C, Karssemeijer N, Platel B. A novel approach to contrast-enhanced breast magnetic resonance imaging for screening: high-resolution ultrafast dynamic imaging. Invest Radiol. 2014. doi:10.1097/RLI.0000000000000057.

18. Wu S, Weinstein SP, DeLeo 3rd MJ, Conant EF, Chen J, Domchek SM, et al. Quantitative assessment of background parenchymal enhancement in breast MRI predicts response to risk-reducing salpingo-oophorectomy: preliminary evaluation in a cohort of BRCA1/2 mutation carriers. Breast Cancer Res BCR. 2015;17(1):67. doi:10.1186/s13058-015-0577-0.

19. King V, Brooks JD, Bernstein JL, Reiner AS, Pike MC, Morris EA. Background parenchymal enhancement at breast MR imaging and breast cancer risk. Radiology. 2011;260(1):50–60. doi:10.1148/radiol.11102156.

20. King V, Goldfarb SB, Brooks JD, Sung JS, Nulsen BF, Jozefara JE, et al. Effect of aromatase inhibitors on background parenchymal enhancement and amount of fibroglandular tissue at breast MR imaging. Radiology. 2012;264(3):670–8. doi:10.1148/radiol.12112669.

21. Pike MC, Pearce CL. Mammographic density, MRI background parenchymal enhancement and breast cancer risk. Ann Oncol Off J Eur Soc Med Oncol/ESMO. 2013;24 Suppl 8:viii37–41. doi:10.1093/annonc/mdt310. PubMed PMID: 24131968; PubMed Central PMCID: PMC3894109.

22. Berg WA, Zhang Z, Lehrer D, Jong RA, Pisano ED, Barr RG, et al. Detection of breast cancer with addition of annual screening ultrasound or a single screening MRI to mammography in women with elevated breast cancer risk. JAMA. 2012;307(13):1394–404. doi:10.1001/jama.2012.388. PubMed PMID: 22474203, PubMed Central PMCID: PMC3891886.

23. Parris T, Wakefield D, Frimmer H. Real world performance of screening breast ultrasound following enactment of Connecticut Bill 458. Breast J. 2013;19(1):64–70. doi:10.1111/tbj.12053.

24. Brem RF, Tabar L, Duffy SW, Inciardi MF, Guingrich JA, Hashimoto BE, et al. Assessing improvement in detection of breast cancer with three-dimensional automated breast US in women with dense breast tissue: the SomoInsight Study. Radiology. 2014;274(3):663–73. doi:10.1148/radiol.14132832.

25. Berg WA, Madsen KS, Schilling K, Tartar M, Pisano ED, Larsen LH, et al. Breast cancer: comparative effectiveness of positron emission mammography and MR imaging in presurgical planning for the ipsilateral breast. Radiology. 2011;258(1):59–72. doi:10.1148/radiol.10100454. PubMed PMID: 21076089, PubMed Central PMCID: PMC3009380.
26. D'Orsi CJ, Sickles EA, Mendelson EB, Morris EA, et al. ACR BI-RADS® Atlas, breast imaging reporting and data system. Reston: American College of Radiology; 2013.
27. Kopans DB. Basic physics and doubts about relationship between mammographically determined tissue density and breast cancer risk. Radiology. 2008;246(2):348–53. doi:10.1148/radiol.2461070309.
28. Sprague BL, Gangnon RE, Burt V, Trentham-Dietz A, Hampton JM, Wellman RD, et al. Prevalence of mammographically dense breasts in the United States. J Nat Cancer Inst. 2014;106(10). doi:10.1093/jnci/dju255. PubMed PMID: 25217577; PubMed Central PMCID: PMC4200066.
29. Wang AT, Vachon CM, Brandt KR, Ghosh K. Breast density and breast cancer risk: a practical review. Mayo Clin Proc. 2014;89(4):548–57.
30. Kolb TM, Lichy J, Newhouse JH. Comparison of the performance of screening mammography, physical examination, and breast US and evaluation of factors that influence them: an analysis of 27,825 patient evaluations. Radiology. 2002;225(1):165–75. doi:10.1148/radiol.2251011667.
31. Boyd NF, Lockwood GA, Byng JW, Tritchler DL, Yaffe MJ. Mammographic densities and breast cancer risk. Cancer Epidemiol Biomark Prev Publ Am Assoc Cancer Res Cospon Am Soc Prev Oncol. 1998;7(12):1133–44.
32. Holm J, Humphreys K, Li J, Ploner A, Cheddad A, Eriksson M, et al. Risk factors and tumor characteristics of interval cancers by mammographic density. J Clin Oncol Off J Am Soc Clin Oncol. 2015;33(9):1030–7. doi:10.1200/JCO.2014.58.9986.
33. Rhodes DJ, Radecki Breitkopf C, Ziegenfuss JY, Jenkins SM, Vachon CM. Awareness of breast density and its impact on breast cancer detection and risk. J Clin Oncol Off J Am Soc Clin Oncol. 2015;33(10):1143–50. doi:10.1200/JCO.2014.57.0325.
34. Yeh VM, Schnur JB, Margolies L, Montgomery GH. Dense breast tissue notification: impact on women's perceived risk, anxiety, and intentions for future breast cancer screening. J Am Coll Radiol JACR. 2015;12(3):261–6. doi:10.1016/j.jacr.2014.11.001. PubMed PMID: 25556313, PubMed Central PMCID: PMC4352389.
35. Trinh L, Ikeda DM, Miyake KK, Trinh J, Lee KK, Dave H, et al. Patient awareness of breast density and interest in supplemental screening tests: comparison of an academic facility and a county hospital. J Am Coll Radiol JACR. 2015;12(3):249–55. doi:10.1016/j.jacr.2014.10.027.
36. Khong KA, Hargreaves J, Aminololama-Shakeri S, Lindfors KK. Impact of the california breast density law on primary care physicians. J Am Coll Radiol JACR. 2015;12(3):256–60. doi:10.1016/j.jacr.2014.09.042.

Chapter 8
Breast Cancer Prevention in Summary

Anna Maria Storniolo and Jill Kremer

Prevention is better than cure. – Desiderius Erasmus (1466–1536)

In a recent consensus statement regarding breast cancer prevention, "preventive therapy" was the new term coined for "chemoprevention" [5]. "Preventive therapy" involves identifying and screening high risk individuals and treating them with therapeutic measures in hopes of decreasing cancer outcomes. This has been compared to the practice in cardiology of screening individuals using serum lipid levels and then treating with statins to prevent cardiovascular events [1].

Applying this to breast cancer is more challenging on several levels. Who should be screened? How should they be treated? Which outcomes are we hoping to change? This is only part of the bigger picture in prevention, which also includes genetic factors, environmental exposures, and lifestyle practices. Adding to further complexity, what is our specific target in breast cancer prevention? Measuring lipids is a simple way to follow a biomarker in the fight against coronary artery disease and related events, but what can serve as a breast cancer biomarker or target for breast cancer prevention? Compounding this problem is that breast cancer is not one single disease, but a collection of malignancies, especially in the case of so-called triple-negative breast cancer [2].

Mammography remains the only recommended imaging tool for breast cancer screening for the general population of women. Randomized clinical trials for women in this age group show that mammography is associated with a 15–20 % relative reduction in breast cancer mortality [3]. However, more recent analyses, including that by Autier et al. [4], point out that the mortality benefit may have been overestimated by the original investigators. A new evaluation of SEER data finds that mammography screening does indeed result in the detection of additional small

A.M. Storniolo, MD (✉) • J. Kremer, MD
IU Simon Cancer Center, Indiana University School of Medicine,
Indianapolis, IN, USA
e-mail: astornio@iu.edu

© Springer International Publishing Switzerland 2016
L.A. Mina et al. (eds.), *Breast Cancer Prevention and Treatment*,
DOI 10.1007/978-3-319-19437-0_8

cancers compared to no screening, but without a concomitant decline in the detection of large cancers, so that ultimately there is no statistically significant difference
in breast cancer mortality [5]. Most recently, the 25-year update of the Canadian
National Breast Screening Study questioned the magnitude of benefit with
mammography screening, especially in areas where adjuvant therapy is readily
available [6]. All of these studies have also pointed to the potential "harms" of
mammography screening, which include radiation exposure, anxiety and emotional
toll from false positives, and overdiagnosis [7].

The differences in conclusions and opinions can be explained in large part by the
understanding that breast cancer is not one disease but a spectrum of diseases with
different biologic behaviors and growth patterns. This reality has enormous
implications with respect to the sensitivity of a given screening modality, as well as
the screening interval. Similarly, not all women have the same risk factors and
therefore may not need to start screening at the same age or undergo it at the same
intervals. The woman most likely to benefit from mammography screening is
someone at high risk, currently defined by family history, certain benign breast his-
tologies, and more recently breast density [8]. With more research, it is hopeful that
biomarkers, genomic profiles, and tissue characteristics will be ways of identifying
women who will benefit from more intense screening and intervention. This
approach, known as "personalized screening," is being actively explored [9].

For the past two decades, efforts have been made to identify women who are at
higher risk for breast cancer [10]. These models can be divided into two categories
of (a) empirical and (b) genetic risk prediction models. These models are limited by
their assumptions about both family inheritance and genetics. They also do not take
into account all risk factors outside of heredity: hormonal, reproductive, mammographic density and benign proliferative disease. Not surprisingly, no model is perfect; each has its own strengths. Amir et al. designed an algorithm according to risk,
assisting in utilizing the best model for the situation. The models include BOADICEA
(the Breast and Ovarian Analysis of Disease Incidence and Carrier Estimation
Algorithm), IBIS (the International Breast Cancer Intervention Study), Claus model,
and Gail model (Fig. 8.1).

Once high-risk individuals have been identified, ideally they will be treated with
preventive therapy that is safe and effective. The drugs currently approved in the
United States for breast cancer risk reduction are the selective estrogen receptor
modulators (SERMs) tamoxifen and raloxifene [23]. Large randomized trials have
also demonstrated the effectiveness of exemestane [11] and anastrozole [12] in this
setting. Other compounds currently being investigated include bisphosphonates,
metformin, statins, COX-2 inhibitors, and fenretinide [13].

Coined by Maximo, Lee, and Jordan, the "ideal" SERM will demonstrate all of the
good effects for aging women and negate the bad. This ideal drug would not only
reduce the risk of breast cancer but also reduce hot flashes, endometrial cancer, osteoporosis, Alzheimer's disease, stroke, and heart disease without the increased risk of
thromboembolic events, decreased libido, and depression [14] (PDR.net) (Fig. 8.2).

Currently, there is no perfect SERM. Tamoxifen carries with it the risk of deep
vein thromboses (DVTs) and increased risk of endometrial cancer [15]. Raloxifene
is approved for osteoporosis and reduces risk of breast cancer in postmenopausal

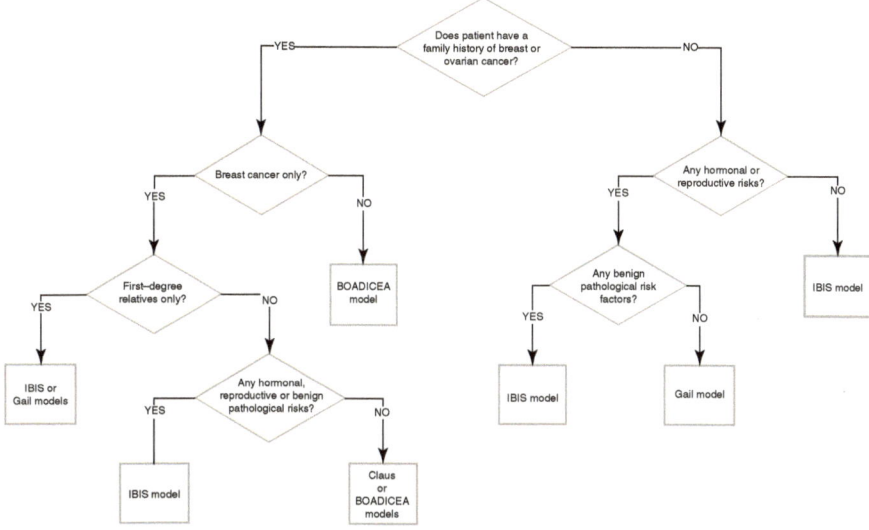

Fig. 8.1 Flowchart for the choice of model for assessing risk of breast cancer over time. *BOADICEA* Breast and Ovarian Analysis of Disease Incidence an Carrier Estimation Algorithm, *IBIS* International Breast Cancer Intervention Study

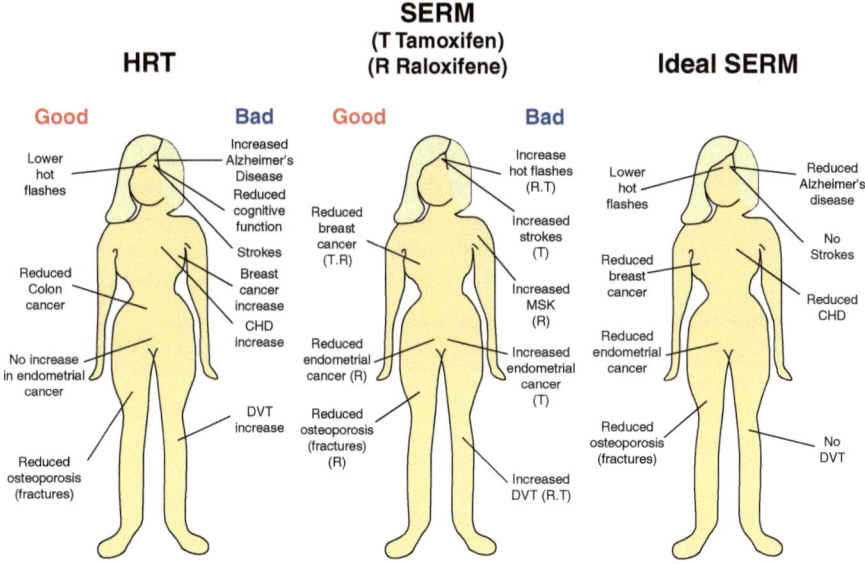

Fig. 8.2 Features of an ideal SERM

women but also shares the risks of venothromboembolic phenomena and hot flushes. Subsequent SERMs are also being studied, with improving side effect profiles. The latest SERM to be approved is ospemifene. With an indication for moderate to severe dyspareunia, it remains to be seen if this drug has any effect in breast cancer risk reduction.

Aromatase inhibitors (AIs) have recently made news as a phase III multicenter trial demonstrated that anastrozole was better than tamoxifen at preventing DCIS transformation into invasive carcinoma in women under the age of 60 years [16]. The biology behind this difference in younger women is not yet understood. This data adds to the growing evidence that estrogen deprivation may be more effective than tamoxifen alone, not only in the adjuvant treatment of invasive breast cancer [17] but also in the postoperative setting of noninvasive breast cancer. When considering the efficacy of aromatase inhibitors for chemoprevention, one must also consider the risks associated with these drugs: osteoporosis, musculoskeletal side effects, and cardiovascular sequelae.

What about modifiable risk factors? Catsburg et al. [18] evaluated 49,613 women via questionnaires on their adherence to the cancer prevention guidelines outlined in the American Cancer Society (ACS) Guidelines on Nutrition and Physical Activity for Cancer Prevention and the World Cancer Research Fund with the American Institute for Cancer Research (WCRF/AICR). These recommendations included BMI goals of 18.5–25, physical activity ≥150–210 min per week, <500 g per week of red and processed meat (<25 g per WCRF), ≥400 g of vegetables and fruits (≥25 g unprocessed grains and legumes per WCRF), whole grain focus per ACS, and ≤1 alcoholic drink per day, and WCRF recommended limiting high calorie foods, sugary drinks, and salt consumption. When women followed all six ACS guidelines, breast cancer was reduced by 31 % compared to those following one guideline or less. This was also seen when six or seven WCRF/AICR guidelines were adhered to. These investigators noted these results paralleled other studies involving dietary modifications. Their data included both premenopausal and postmenopausal women. In a summary by Harvie et al. [19] published in the ASCO educational book, the authors reviewed the evidence of breast cancer risk reduction linked to reduced body fat and alcohol consumption in the cancer prevention guidelines, in postmenopausal women with less dietary effect.

In a randomized controlled trial by Friedenreich et al [20], the investigators were able to demonstrate that in postmenopausal women, moderate to vigorous exercise for 300 min/week was better than 150 min/week in reducing BMI and thus breast cancer risk. It is hypothesized that activity decreases cancer risk by reducing "endogenous sex hormone concentrations, insulin resistance and chronic low-grade inflammation [19]."

Yet, with all the modalities mentioned above, the result has been decreased incidence of breast cancer, but so far no decrease in mortality. This is possibly secondary to lag time, confounding factors, and identification of high-risk individuals.

Perhaps our most glaring barrier in preventing breast cancer resides in our lack of understanding of the enemy. Yet how can we understand breast cancer if we do not understand the normal breast? The normal female breast is probably the most inherently dynamic of all of our organs. Throughout a woman's life, the breast undergoes multiple physiologic changes—childhood, puberty, pregnancy, lactation, involution, and menopause. Even within the same month, the breast changes with the phases of the menstrual cycle. All of these changes are regulated through finely tuned molecular

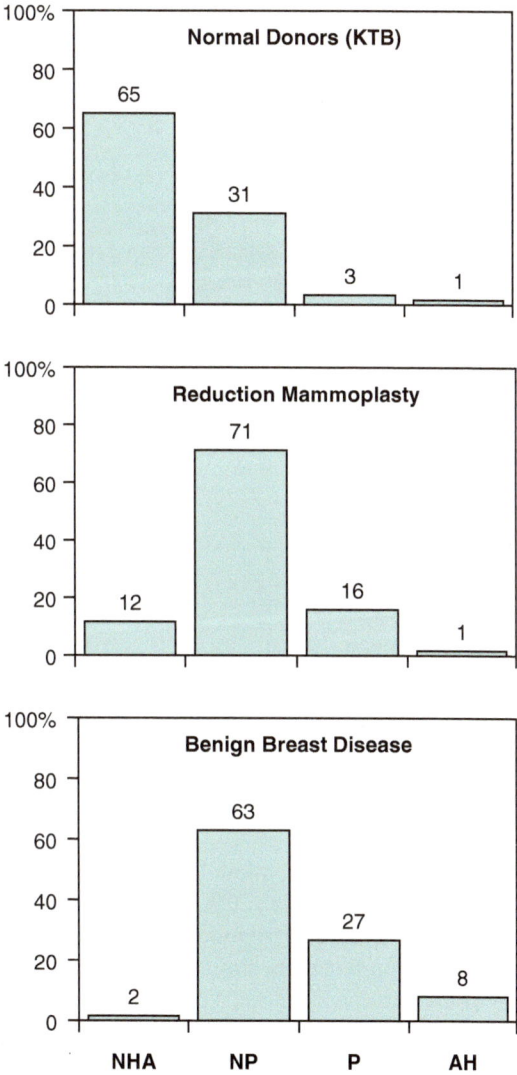

Fig. 8.3 Histologic findings in normal breast tissues: comparison to reduction mammoplasty and benign breast disease tissues. *NHA* no histologic abnormality; *NP* non proliferative disease; *P* proliferative disease; *AH* atypical hyperplasia

"switches." It stands to reason that if we better understood these switches, we would gain an understanding of how and why they malfunction. These regulatory "misfires" are the basis of breast oncogenesis. In other words, if we understood *normal*, we would better understand *abnormal*, or cancer, and then be able to interfere.

Previous studies involving "normal breast tissue" actually were plagued by availability. Tissue was obtained from women who were already undergoing biopsy for suspicion of cancer, from remnants of reduction mammoplasty or from tissue surrounding cancerous findings (so-called adjacent normal) [21, 22]. Degnim et al. demonstrated that samples from women with benign breast disease and reduction mammoplasty are not even histologically normal (Fig. 8.3).

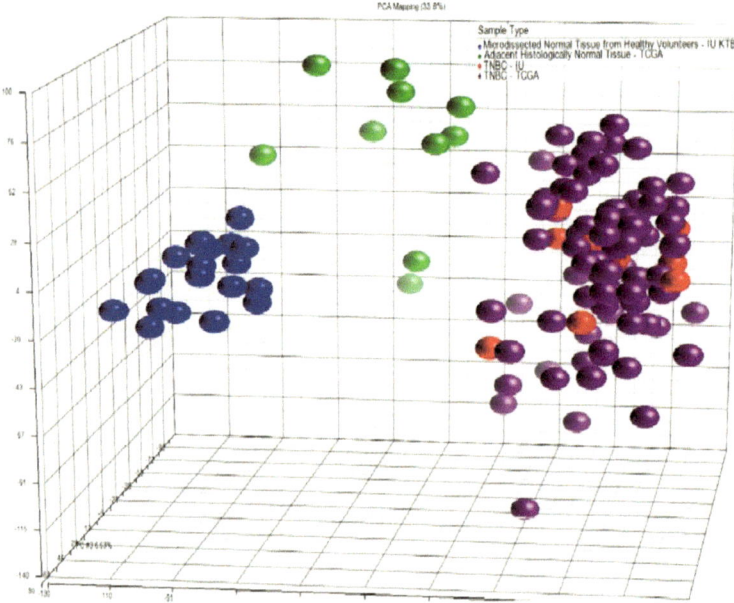

Fig. 8.4 Unsupervised principal components analysis (PCA) of 14,271 expressed genes demonstrating global gene expression differences between microdissected normal tissue from healthy volunteers, adjacent histologically normal tissue, and triple-negative breast cancers. The sample types cluster into three distinct groups with the TNBCs from IU and from the TCGA clustering together, demonstrating effective merging of the data. *IU* indiana university; *KTB* Susan G. Komen Tissue Bank at the Indiana University Simon Cancer Center; *TCGA* The Cancer Genome Atlas

Radovich et al. explored this question at a molecular level in the Principal Components Analysis (PCA) shown in Fig. 8.4, showing that "adjacent normal" (green) is in fact quite distinct from tissue obtained from healthy women volunteers (blue) and in fact more similar to frank malignancy (purple and red) (Fig. 8.4).

Research has been geared toward analyzing cancer, evaluating mutations, and discovering genomic signatures of malignancy. Yet how do we really understand them without a molecular understanding of the normal breast?

It is always the simple that produces the marvelous. – Amelia Barr (1831–1919)

Availability of reliable sources of normal tissue has been a problem until recently. The Susan G. Komen Tissue Bank at the Indiana University Simon Cancer Center was created in response to the 1998 National Cancer Institute Breast Cancer Review Group that identified our limited understanding of the normal mammary gland as a deficiency needing to be addressed in order to move forward in our advancements in breast cancer:

Our limited understanding of the biology and developmental genetics of the normal mammary gland is a barrier to progress. Much of our biological research in breast cancer has focused on understanding the initiation and development of the disease. This research has been fruitful, but it is now clear that a more complete understanding of the normal mammary gland at each stage of development—from infancy through adulthood—will be a critical underpinning of continued advances in detecting, preventing and treating breast cancer. This focus represents a major shift in breast biology research and requires increased support for these studies and the materials needed to conduct them.

Founded in 2007 at Indiana University, the KTB is currently an international resource for normal breast tissue gathered from healthy women volunteers. The only one of its kind, the KTB serves as a repository of breast tissue and blood, including extensive health histories of thousands of donors. It also uniquely serves as a "virtual tissue bank" to assist in building upon earlier research results, facilitating accelerated data dissemination.

As we learn more about normal breast tissue and its complex "life cycle," we will hopefully uncover more biomarkers which can serve as indicators of risk and/or targets for prevention. As personalized medicine develops, vaccinations will be a consideration. Drs. Stanton and Disis of the Tumor Vaccine Group at the University of Washington discussed in an editorial the possibilities afforded in learning more about the immune environment of breast cancer. Type 1 T helper cells (Th1) help facilitate an antitumor response, and there is current evidence that specific epitopes of this type used in a multiantigen vaccine can prevent breast cancer in mice. Clinical trials will be soon testing this in women [22].

It is through continued persistence and determination that the pursuit of complete prevention is sought. Ideally it will allow us to identify those at high risk and mitigate the development of breast carcinoma, all the while decreasing the risk of harm and keeping societal costs low. Prevention is a sport in endurance, and we all will continue running this marathon in pursuit of a cure.

Someone is sitting in the shade today because someone planted a tree a long time ago. – Warren Buffett

References

1. Baigent C, Keech A, Kearney PM, Blackwell L, Buck G, Pollicino C, et al. Efficacy and safety of cholesterol-lowering treatment: prospective meta-analysis of data from 90,056 participants in 14 randomised trials of statins. Lancet. 2005;366:1267–78.
2. Radovich M, Clare SE, Atale R, Pardo I, Hancock BA, Solzak JP, et al. Characterizing the heterogeneity of triple-negative breast cancers using microdissected normal ductal epithelium and RNA-sequencing. Breast Cancer Res Treat. 2014;143(1):57–68.
3. Nelson HD, Tyne K, Naik A, Bougatsos C, Chan BK, Humphrey L. Screening for breast cancer: an update for the U.S. Preventive services task force. Ann Intern Med. 2009;151: 727–37.
4. Autier P, Boniol M, Smans M, Sullivan R, Boyle P. Statistical analyses in Swedish randomized trials on mammography screening and in other randomized trials on cancer screening: a systematic review. J R Soc Med. 2015;108(11):440-50.
5. Harding C, Pompei F, Burmistrov D, Welch G, Abebe R, Wilson R. Breast cancer screening, incidence, and mortality across US counties. JAMA Intern Med. 2015;175(9):1483–9. Online publication 7/6/2015.
6. Miller AB, Wall C, Baines CJ, Sun P, To T, Narod SA. Twenty five year follow-up for breast cancer incidence and mortality of the Canadian National Breast Screening Study: randomised screening trial. BMJ. 2014;348:g366.

7. Koleva-Kolarova RG, Zhan Z, Greuter MJW, Feenstra TL, De Bock GH. Simulation models in population breast cancer screening: a systematic review. Breast. 2015;24:354–63.

8. McCormack VA, dos Santos Silva I. Breast density and parenchymal patterns as markers of breast cancer risk: a meta-analysis. Cancer Epidemiol Biomarkers Prev. 2006;15:1159–69.

9. Onega T, Beaber EF, Sprague BL, Barlow WE, Haas JS, Tosteson ANA, Schnall MD, Armstrong K, Schapira MM, Geller B, Weaver DL, Conant EF. Breast cancer screening in an era of personalized regimens. Cancer. 2014;120:2955–64.

10. Amir E, Freedman OC, Seruga B, Evans DG. Assessing women at high risk of breast cancer: a review of risk assessment models. J Natl Cancer Inst. 2010;102(10):680–91.

11. Goss PE, Ingle JN, Alés-Martínez JE, NCIC CTG MAP.3 Study investigators. Exemestane for breast-cancer prevention in postmenopausal women. N Engl J Med. 2011;364(25):2381–91.

12. Cuzick J, Sestak I, Forbes JF, Dowsett M, Knox J, Cawthorn S, Saunders C, Roche N, Mansel RE, von Minckwitz G, Bonanni B, Palva T, Howell A, IBIS-II investigators. Anastrozole for prevention of breast cancer in high-risk postmenopausal women (IBIS-II): an international, double-blind, randomised placebo-controlled trial. Lancet. 2014;383:1041–8.

13. Cuzick J, DeCensi A, Arun B, Brown PH, Castiglione M, Dunn B, Forbes JF, Glaus A, Howell A, von Minckwitz G, Vogel V, Zwierzina H. Preventative therapy for breast cancer: a consensus statement. Lancet Oncol. 2011;12:496–503.

14. Maximov PY, Lee TM, Jordan VC. The discovery and development of selective estrogen receptor modulators (SERMs) for clinical practice. Curr Clin Pharmacol. 2013;8:135–55.

15. Tamoxifendrugsummary.http://www.pdr.net/drug-summary/tamoxifen-citrate?druglabelid=664. Accessed 12 Aug 2015.

16. Margolese RG, Cecchini RS, Julian TB, et al. Primary results, NRG Oncology/NSABP B-35: a clinical trial of anastrozole (A) versus tamoxifen (tam) in postmenopausal patients with DCIS undergoing lumpectomy plus radiotherapy. J Clin Oncol. 2015;33(suppl): abstr LBA500.

17. Pagani O, Regan MM, Walley BA, et al. Adjuvant exemestane with ovarian suppression in premenopausal breast cancer. N Engl J Med. 2014;371:107–18.

18. Catsburg C, Miller AB, Rohan TE. Adherence to cancer prevention guidelines and risk of breast cancer. Int J Cancer. 2014;135:2444–52.

19. Harvie M, Howell A, Evans DG. Can diet and lifestyle prevent breast cancer: what is the evidence? ASCO Educ Book. 2015:e66–73.

20. Friedenreich CM, Neilson HK, O'Reilly R, Duha A, Yasui Y, Morielli AR, Adams SC, Courneya KS. Effects of a high vs moderate volume of aerobic exercise on adiposity outcomes in postmenopausal women. JAMA Oncol. 2015;1(6):766–76. Online publication 7/16/2015.

21. Degnim AC, Visscher DW, Hoskin TL, Frost MH, Vierkant RA, Vachon CM, et al. Histologic findings in normal breast tissues: comparison to reduction mammoplasty and benign breast disease tissues. Breast Cancer Res Treat. 2012;133(1):169–77.

22. Sherman ME, Figurroa JD, Henry JE, Clare SE, Rufenbarger C, The SAM, Susan G. Komen for the Cure Tissue Bank at the IU Simon Cancer Center: a unique resource for defining the "molecular histology" of the breast. Cancer Prev Res. 2012;5:528–35.

23. Stanton SE, Disis ML. Designing vaccines to prevent cancer recurrence or invasive disease. Immunotherapy. 2015;7(2):69–72. Editorial.

Index

© Springer International Publishing Switzerland 2016
L.A. Mina et al. (eds.), *Breast Cancer Prevention and Treatment*,
DOI 10.1007/978-3-319-19437-0